C000218689

RAPID RESPONSE

Dedication

This book is dedicated to Nicole, Dawn and Kyle, two daughters and a son whose quality time was most affected.

RAPID RESPONSE

My inside story as a motor racing life-saver

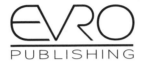

Dr Stephen Olvey

FOREWORD BY ALEX ZANARDI
AFTERWORD BY DARIO FRANCHITTI

© Stephen Olvey 2019

All rights reserved. No part of this publication may be reproduced or stored in a retrieval system or transmitted, in any form or by any means, electronic, mechanical, photocopying, recording or otherwise, without prior permission in writing from Evro Publishing.

Published by Haynes in hardback in April 2006
Published by Haynes in paperback (with new material) in December 2011
Published by Evro in hardback (with further new material) in April 2019

ISBN 978-1-910505-39-7

Published by Evro Publishing, Westrow House, Holwell, Sherborne, Dorset DT9 5LF, UK

www.evropublishing.com

Jacket illustration by James Gibson
Jacket design by Richard Parsons

Printed and bound in Slovenia by GPS Group

Author's note
The events and issues portrayed in this book are as I remember them – others may remember them in a slightly different way.

ACKNOWLEDGEMENTS

Robin Miller, race driver, journalist, and friend.

Gordon Kirby, respected motorsports journalist who graciously translated Alex Zanardi's heartfelt Foreword into English.

Professor Sid Watkins, good friend, visionary, superb neurosurgeon and dogged compatriot in our quest to advance medicine and safety in motorsport.

Dr. Terry Trammell, good friend and cherished colleague through times both good and bad as well as everything else we have managed to get ourselves into.

Dan Boyd, consummate racing photographer who always seems to capture the right moment.

Indianapolis Motor Speedway, the world's premier racing facility, for its provision of photographs of days long past.

The nurses, medics, firemen and track workers who work tirelessly in the volatile world of auto racing, and who spend their time with little in the way of reward so that the rest of us can enjoy the world's most spectacular spectator sport.

CONTENTS

FOREWORD BY
ALEX ZANARDI

During the course of life, it happens that one looks back and realizes that some particular events have transformed themselves into great opportunities.

I decided to become a professional racecar driver because of my passion for cars and racing and I believe I've been very fortunate in my choice. I am convinced of this, because in order to succeed in such a difficult and competitive sport like auto racing, talent, hard work and sacrifices are never enough. Passion is what pushes you along as you fight to make it, and passion is actually what turns everyday struggles into a fantastic adventure.

Behind the short-lived emotions that a racecar driver experiences on a Sunday afternoon when you see the checkered flag and win a race, there is an adolescence that differs from that of your pals. There is less discothèque time and fewer nights out with friends, and more time spent training and going to bed early in order to be in perfect shape for the next race.

One has to endure failure, doors closed in your face, and stupid mistakes that, with hindsight, you vow not to repeat. However, these elements are the keys to success because they test your passion in such a way that they either break or strengthen you in a permanent way.

During this journey, regardless of how bumpy it may be, a racecar driver has the fortune of practicing what he really loves and the preparation for that special Sunday becomes, perhaps, the most passionate part of the job.

But what happens if the long-awaited dream never

materializes? What are you left with? Some people, who face this dilemma, choose not to undertake the tasks and instead choose safer roads and perhaps they are right. But what they forgo is a chance to chase their dream.

I believe this is true for many professional fields where people don't aspire to become a racecar driver, and I believe the analogy is particularly true for the medical profession.

The profession of a doctor, in order to be successful, necessarily needs to be fulfilled with passion, courage, meticulous training and a great sense of responsibility.

For the doctors, who well know they provide a vital contribution to their job, there is a constant interior conflict between their patients and their families and friends who inevitably undergo the effects of the sacrifices doctors go through in order to practice their duty.

'Rapid Response' doctors have to feel they are on a mission, they have to have this burning passion that makes them overcome obstacles and hardships. Otherwise they would have chosen to practice in a much more ambulatory environment.

Although there are similarities there is also a substantial difference between a racecar driver and a 'Rapid Response' doctor. When a driver wins his race he is in the spotlight, goes on the podium, fans adore him and he gets to be interviewed on TV. The doctor, on the other hand, is always ready to win his race, but hopes that he never needs to compete because he knows that this would coincide with the misfortune of someone else.

On the 15th of September 2001 I am sure that my friend Dr. Steve Olvey wished he never raced that day. He would have loved not to show the world his medical talent and the fast thinking that he demonstrated in saving my life.

I know that Dr. Olvey and Dr. Terry Trammell would have liked to have spent another afternoon just watching the race on the TV screens at the medical center, in the shadows of their heroes who were racing. I know they would have loved for me to finish the last 13 laps and seen my signature 'doughnuts' as a testament to my victory during that difficult season.

As a driver, I never really fully understood the importance of the difficult responsibility of my medical heroes until destiny chose to place my life in their hands. Frankly, I am glad that these hands were those of Dr. Steve, Dr. Terry, and of the whole Safety Team that was working during those years.

I admit that each time I arrived at a track, my worries were to go to the garage and check out the racecar, talk to the engineers and mechanics, circle the track on my scooter in order to understand its secrets. But it never crossed my mind to go to the medical center in order to understand those kinds of details in case I ever needed them. Maybe it's because, like all drivers, I was born too optimistic to worry about such things.

I believe that all the people who silently looked after our safety with incredible modesty (and never for monetary reasons, I assure you), were carrying out their 'mission' motivated by passion for their job and for racing, and by human kindness, rather than simply because of wanting to do a good job.

I also believe that Dr. Olvey, as Medical Director of the series, started to save my life long before I even realized it. He instituted the practice of selecting the finest hospitals around the race tracks, so that he and his team could make vital decisions in split seconds, should a situation arise, without delegating critical decisions to the local staff as happens in other sports. I know this for a fact. I truly believe that these procedures, along with the training and discipline of each member of the Safety Team, were the difference between life and death in my accident.

There is no measure for the love and passion that doctors like Steve Olvey put into their work, and in a way it's sad to think that they get recognition only during tragic circumstances. One has to remember that doctors are human beings with feelings. They have an uncanny ability to set aside feelings and emotions during their delicate work, but if the patient who suffers is a friend, the doctor suffers with him.

When I was skiing in Beaver Creek last winter it was made

clear to me how much Dr. Olvey suffered on September 15, 2001. It was clear because there I was skiing, despite having lost both legs, but not my spirit and good mood, and I saw him overcome by emotion. In those tears of emotion I saw much more than any words can ever describe.

My Dad always told me that in order to go home at night and like what you see in the mirror, winning was not important, but trying your best to win surely was. I truly believe this.

In May of 2003, as a disabled person, I returned to the Lausitzring, the track where my accident occurred, to complete those last 13 laps which I didn't manage to complete a year and a half earlier. A lot of people called this feat 'heroic'. But honestly, I just had fun!

When Dr. Olvey saw me going around the track at my 'usual' pace, in search of the limit like nothing had happened and not just cruising around, hopefully he viewed my ordeal in a different light, positively that is.

I would like to think that he understands that what I still have in life, thanks to him, is much more than what I have lost.

I would like to think and hope that on that day, on top of having recognized the status of Dr. Olvey and of all the Safety Team's success, I also helped all my family and friends to achieve closure on that chapter of our life.

But most of all, I would like to think that Dr. Olvey and his team's hard work, long hours, dedication, their gypsy life and most of all the time away from their families, was not spent in vain. I, for one, will always be thankful.

And if one night at home, Steve, you look in the mirror and you like what you see, it means only one thing – that you have good eyes!

Caro Amico, ti abbraccio.

PREFACE
GERMANY 2001

Raceday dawned gray and dreary with a distinct threat of rain. More than 80,000 spectators found their way into the ultra-modern race track located about a mile from the *autobahn* connecting Berlin and Dresden. Closer to Dresden, the track lay neatly organized next to the small town of Klettwitz, and had been christened the Lausitzring Eurospeedway. We had arrived for the race early and were watching the opening ceremonies get underway. They would become the most touching and meaningful I had ever seen. It was hard to believe Dresden had been on the wrong side of the Berlin wall just 12 years before.

The procession unfolding before us included some very tough-looking former communist policemen and firemen. They were marching in uniform holding tiny American flags. German schoolchildren marched behind them dressed surprisingly as American pioneers, many with large, genuine tears wetting their ruddy cheeks. Our brightly uniformed crewmen were lined up soldier-like behind their respective racecars. Each of them soon alternated hand-in-hand with the German officers as the band played the American national anthem. Only 12 years since the despair and desolation behind the Iron Curtain, it was truly unbelievable!

The race was now less than an hour away. Alex Zanardi was going through his pre-race ritual. The other 25 drivers were doing the same. Each with a different set of habits and superstitions developed over years of competition. Some still feared the color green, some would dress in a certain order, left glove always on before the right one. All the drivers were in final preparation for the grueling and dangerous 500-kilometer test of strength and endurance that lay ahead.

The pageant slowly drew to a close with Scottish pipers playing a mournful rendition of *Amazing Grace*. Most of those gathered were, by now, in tears. The poignant display had been hastily, but beautifully put together in response to the horrible events of September 11, 2001. The day we landed in Dresden.

My wife Lynne and I, along with my good friend and associate Dr. Terry Trammell and his wife Rhonda, found out about the terrorist attacks shortly after we arrived at our hotel three days before the race. We had flown from Miami to Frankfurt and then on to Dresden for Championship Auto Racing Teams' first race in Germany. Terry and I had been working races together since 1984. He was CART's Chief Orthopedic Consultant and I was their Director of Medical Affairs. The two of us had dedicated our adult lives to treating and preventing injuries to racecar drivers.

Following check-in, we were approached by a very apprehensive CART official. He told us in near hysterics that a plane had just crashed into the World Trade Center in New York. My first thought was that some pilot had really screwed up! The four of us rushed to our rooms to catch CNN. Lynne reached the TV first and flipped it on just in time to see the second plane crash into the remaining tower. Stunned, we both sat down in absolute silence.

CNN abruptly switched cameras to reveal an additional crash site in Pennsylvania, followed quickly by the scene of havoc around the crumbled wall at the Pentagon. What on earth was happening? It appeared that our government was systematically being attacked and destroyed while we were stuck in Germany, 4,000 miles away.

The first thing that came to my mind was the safety of the rest of our family. Our three children and three grandchildren were in the United States. Where were they? Were they okay? Why did this happen? Why are we over here now for Christ's sake?

"Assholes!"

I didn't know what else to say.

"Cocksuckers!"

My vocabulary is very limited at times like this.

Lynne sat in stunned silence.

"Oh my God!" she finally replied.

The two of us were paralyzed, helpless to know what to do next. There was this tremendous urge to flee. But where would we go? All flights to the U.S. had been canceled. We tried to make a call. All phone lines were busy. We were stuck! Thankfully, after another hour or so it appeared the attacks were over, at least for the time being. We hastily showered, changed clothes, and headed for the hotel lobby. We certainly had no desire to be by ourselves!

The lobby was packed with people. The hotel staff had thoughtfully placed a big TV just outside of the bar and everyone was sitting or standing around it still in disbelief. Dave Hollander, a burly fireman who drives one of CART's four Safety Trucks, was wandering around aimlessly, his face despairingly pale. His daughter, we learned, worked in Building One of the World Trade Center. He was a wreck. No answer on his daughter's cell phone, no service, no way to call out at all.

The hotel allowed dinner to be served anywhere in the lobby so most of us tried to eat something. Vodka seemed to be the best answer for the moment. Around seven o'clock German time Hollander finally heard from his daughter. Luckily, she had kept her morning dental appointment just a few blocks from her office. With that good news everyone began eating in earnest for the first time since breakfast. We loosened up a little and managed to survive the night. Anger and hostility remained the predominant emotions.

The next morning Terry and I headed for the race track as we had been doing for the past 20 years. Lynne and Rhonda were with us. Flights to the U.S. were still grounded so it became business as usual. The four of us were awash in a wide variety of emotions, but we still had a job to do. We headed on to the *autobahn*.

Reportedly, the track was only 30 miles from our hotel. I drove the rental car while Terry served as my navigator. The wives jumped into the back seat. Bad deal! Terry and I could get lost trying to find our way out of a two-room house. Years before, *en route* to one of our races in Portland, Oregon, the two of us had been driving for a suspiciously long time after leaving the airport. We were trying to find our assigned hotel, supposedly in Portland. When we sailed past a sign on the Interstate reading: 'Seattle 10 miles' we realized we had really screwed up. Our sense of direction had not improved much in the ensuing years as we managed to get within 14 miles of the Polish border. Screaming voices from the back seat finally convinced us to turn around. We had driven more than 100 miles out of our way.

When we finally did reach the track, we were surprised to find such a beautiful facility. The slightly banked two-mile oval had been built entirely on speculation. Former East Germany still had over 20% unemployment. In addition to the oval, there was a seven-mile road course and a second, larger oval that was used primarily for testing. Debt service on a facility that size was phenomenal!

The mood at the track was somber, as expected. Everyone was robotically going through the motions required to put on a CART event. Terry and I were no exception. We began our search for the infield medical center. A large Red Cross flag identified the facility. It was very German; simple, functional, clean, and extremely well equipped. What a change from the early days! I had arranged for all of the necessary life-saving equipment to be in place well in advance of our arrival. Thanks to the German medics I was able to duplicate what we have in our mobile medical unit back home. It would have been cost-prohibitive to move our own stuff to another continent.

In preparing for the German race, I had neglected one thing. None of the German doctors spoke a lick of English. This was a major oversight! Fortunately, the daughter of one of their physicians spoke perfect English. I quickly appointed her chief translator. If something bad were to happen, we needed the ability to communicate rapidly and effectively with our German partners.

We carefully unloaded our supplies. These consisted primarily of specialized orthopedic splints and some popular over-the-counter drugs not available in Europe in a form familiar to most of us Americans. We also carried equipment used by our trainers that was no different than what any other traveling sports team might carry. Once settled in, we began to get acquainted with our German hosts. Without exception, all of the Germans on the medical staff were extremely friendly, and very empathetic to what had happened to America the day before.

The helicopter crew arrived on schedule, always a worry for me until they actually appear on site. Unlike several past experiences in other countries, the Germans provided us with everything they had promised. We had state-of-the-art cardiac and blood pressure monitors, the latest German ventilator, blood warming devices, fluoroscopy, a movie version of X-ray as well as conventional X-ray, and a complete operating room suite with anesthesia. We were equipped to handle any life-threatening emergency that might present itself. At least that's what we thought. We numbly dug in for the event, still working mostly by remote control.

Late in the day Joe Heitzler, CART's latest in a long line of CEOs, surprisingly told us there might not be a race. All sporting events in the States had been cancelled, as had most shows and concerts in response to the terrorist attacks. CART was in a real jam. If they ran the race as scheduled, people back home might not understand. If they didn't run the race, several thousand Germans would be even less understanding. The cities of Berlin and Dresden stood to lose hundreds of thousands of tourist dollars and the track, that was on shaky ground to begin with, would gravely suffer financially as well. It was the proverbial *Catch 22*. We were the largest contingent of Americans overseas at the time of the attacks, and potentially vulnerable ourselves.

Heitzler hastily met with the American ambassador and several prominent German officials. They came up with the perfect solution. The event would be held as a memorial to all who had perished in the heinous attacks of 9/11. Bowing down to the terrorists was exactly what the terrorists wanted people to do. The name of the race was promptly changed to 'The German Memorial' and was scheduled to go off as planned.

Largely due to the overwhelming friendliness of the German people, most of us really began to enjoy being over there. We all fell in love with the city of Dresden. To think that we virtually destroyed the place with firebombs during the Second World War was inconceivable. Charred remains still stained most of the downtown buildings, providing a grim reminder of how sick and depraved war is.

At night candles glowed in building after building, symbolizing the strong sympathy the Germans felt toward the U.S. Strangers would walk up and pat you on the back, look you straight in the eye, and graciously tell you they were sorry. I doubt seriously if we would have treated them the same way had they been the ones so viciously attacked.

Jon Potter, a long-time friend and director of the Championship Drivers Association, along with Father Phil De Rea, our traveling priest, discovered, as always, the best restaurants in town. Both of them set their clocks around mealtimes and made it a point to locate the gastronomical havens of the cities we visited. We ate well, found some good wines, and began to relax a little during the days leading up to the race.

Only minutes remained now before the start. Ever darkening clouds had enveloped the Speedway. The mood in the grandstands nonetheless was one of festive anticipation and national pride as the 'German Memorial' was about to get underway.

Zanardi, two-time CART champion, had just returned to our series following a lackluster year in Formula One in 1999. He had followed that up with a year of spectating in 2000. He had been struggling for most of the current season with no podium finishes to show for his efforts. Many knowledgeable participants thought his career as a competitive driver might just be over. Never one to give up, Alex climbed into his car thinking today might bring him that elusive first victory of the year.

In the preceding race, he had begun to drive like the old Zanardi. When he left CART in 1999 to compete in Formula One, he was easily CART's most popular driver. He was best known for his spectacular passes. He would often pass other drivers in areas never before thought possible. Like the time he took to the dirt in order to pass a bewildered Bryan Herta for the win at the top of the famous Corkscrew in Laguna Seca. Alex would never quit trying. He would frequently come from behind against overwhelming odds, passing everybody to win a race long after he had been written off. In Germany, he finally seemed to have regained his old competitiveness. Alex, it seemed, was back.

As he climbed into his car, cheers for Zanardi could be heard above the noise that surrounds the start of every race. A determined Alex, waving to the delight of the crowd, drove out of the pits and into formation for the parade lap. Several of his friends had traveled from nearby Italy to watch him race. They did this in spite of the fact that Formula One's Italian Grand Prix was being held on the same weekend.

It was still cold and windy with rain threatening when the command was given to start engines. My usual pre-race apprehension consumed me as I tried to anticipate what might happen. Terry and I were always more apprehensive on the oval tracks in spite of the fact that two of our last three fatalities had occurred on road courses. Speeds were generally much higher on the ovals and there was nowhere to go but into a solid concrete wall if you lost control.

Potter settled in with me in the care center along with our two nurses, Sue Dunham and Liz Friede. Terry was in Safety 2, a bright yellow Toyota rescue truck equipped with necessary advanced life-support paraphernalia, stationed just inside of Turn 3. He would be the physician at the scene of any incident on the race track. It would be his job to address any immediate life-threatening injuries. Lynne was working in the pits as a spotter for ESPN, the popular cable sports network in the United States. Rhonda was driving for the Pace Car Team. I confirmed that the helicopter could fly safely in the low-hanging overcast.

The race started with all 80,000 spectators on their feet. Those of us confined to the care center gathered around the TV monitor. Our firemen and paramedics that made up the Simple Green Safety Team were in their respective vehicles, poised and ready to handle anything the drivers threw their way. I rechecked my checklist.

The race progressed without incident. Almost immediately, Zanardi began to move up from his 22nd starting position. He tore through the field. Like a fighter pilot tracking 'bogies' he was reeling in, and passing, the other drivers one by one. The crowd jumped to their feet, cheering wildly, when he gained the lead late in the race. With 13 laps remaining, he had one more stop to make for fuel. Stopping would cause him to relinquish that lead but he had no choice and headed for the pits.

Lynne, with ESPN reporter Gary Gerould, ran to Alex's pit just as he pulled in. It was like '97 and '98: Alex was in the hunt! The pit stop took less than 12 seconds. Waved back out by his crewman, Alex floored his maroon-colored racecar, engulfing the entire pit area in blue smoke, spinning his tires as he rejoined the race. He was determined to regain the lead.

He charged out of the pits and on to the exit road leading back to the racing surface. At this track, as at many oval tracks, the pit exit road runs parallel to the racing surface, separated by only a thin strip of grass as it parallels Turns 1 and 2. A gentle merge back on to the race track occurs at the entrance to the backstretch. Ominously, no guardrail separates the pit road from the racing surface.

As Zanardi entered the portion of pit road that parallels the first turn he was going way too fast. Losing traction, the rear end of his car suddenly slid sideways. The car then shot backward on to the thin grassy strip, its rear wheels leaving the ground as it bounced on to the race track directly into the path of the two Player's Team cars closing at over 190 mph. Patrick Carpentier, driving the first of them, missed Zanardi's car by only a few inches. Alex Tagliani's car, running immediately behind Carpentier, had nowhere else to go and slammed into Zanardi, piercing his car broadside. Both cars exploded into a zillion pieces. The nose of Tagliani's speared Zanardi's cockpit just below and in front of his pelvis. Alex's car was torn open in a spray of shrapnel. Bits of carbon fibre, along with hundreds of small metal fragments, were propelled in every direction. Razor sharp pieces ripped into his legs, shredding the tissue and fracturing bones in the process. The force of the impact caused an eruption of debris that resembled a bomb-blast. Pieces of Alex's legs were showered over the entire second turn.

I watched the TV monitor in horror, fearing the worst. I was sure no-one could survive that kind of an impact. I was convinced we had just witnessed our first double fatality. Zanardi's Reynard ground to a stop in the middle of the track, halfway through Turn 2. The front of the car was gone. The first safety truck arrived within 19 seconds. I watched helplessly from the medical center as our medics quickly stabilized Alex's neck and carefully removed his helmet. His breathing was obstructed and he was unconscious. Blood spewed from both legs. Both femoral arteries, the large ones that carry all the blood to the legs, had been severed. One of our medics manually cleared his airway and his breathing improved. A small tube, designed to keep the upper airway open, was inserted through his nose.

The second safety truck, with Dr. Trammell on board, arrived within seconds of the first. Tagliani's car had come to rest at the top of the track just downstream from Zanardi's; he was being ignored. All the attention was focused on the rapidly exsanguinating 35-year-old Italian.

Terry leapt from his truck, slipping and falling almost immediately. He was able to claw his way over the bizarre mix of blood and racing fluids as he finally reached Alex, slumped unconscious in what was left of his car. Terry knew there wasn't much time left. Zanardi had lost most of his blood volume in the one to two minutes that had elapsed since the crash. The bloody scene around the car was testament to that.

Terry yelled frantically for more wound dressings as he packed the right stump to control the deluge. He then turned his attention to the left leg that was severed much higher than the right. The left femoral artery was spewing blood like a faucet. Michael Andretti would later remark that when Alex's car was spinning down the track it looked like a big lawn sprinkler. The large veins also bled severely. Heavy packing and pressure hadn't stopped the hemorrhage.

Thinking fast, Terry jerked a belt off one of our paramedics to make a tourniquet. He wrapped it tightly around the stump, but it slipped off. He put it back on, tighter this time. It seemed to stem the flow of blood, at least for the time being. I continued to wait helplessly for a report.

The Safety Team carefully lifted Zanardi from the remains of the car and placed him in the waiting ambulance. His neck was supported in a collar and his back was stabilized on a backboard. The bleeding had slowed somewhat, but both legs continued to ooze.

In the care center, I had already notified the flight crew to get ready. The injuries were so severe it didn't make sense to waste time inside the care center. We would stabilize him at the helicopter and send him on to the trauma center without an unnecessary and potentially deadly delay and transfer. I knew he was bleeding from more than just his legs. Internally, any number of injuries may have occurred. After what seemed like an eternity, Terry finally called me on our private radio channel.

"This is bad Steve, really bad! Both legs are gone."

"Can anything be salvaged?"

"No, there's nothing left. His legs are in pieces!"

The ambulance careened into the landing zone. I ran out to meet it as the doors flew open. Terry, blood soaked, burst from the vehicle looking like he had been shot. We struggled to get Alex to the waiting helicopter. There, I examined him along with

21

the German physician. His breathing was extremely labored, threatening to stop altogether. His skin was ashen. There was no movement. His eyes had rolled to the back of his head and were glassy and empty. His pulse was barely detectable. He was dying.

We quickly placed a tube in Alex's windpipe and began to breathe for him, using a rubber bag. Simultaneously, a German medic placed him on a heart monitor and applied an oxygen sensor to his finger. His oxygen level was dangerously low. His blood pressure started to drop rapidly and his heartbeat had become irregular and barely detectable. We had to work fast.

He needed fluid to replace the lost blood. We rapidly inserted three large catheters into the veins of his arms and began running a saline solution in as fast as it would flow. With the fluid, his blood pressure began a slow rise. Soon his heart rhythm stabilized. His oxygen level rose to an acceptable level now that his airway was secure. I told the helicopter to leave for Berlin, 60 miles away. The entire rescue had taken less than 15 minutes.

Before the weekend, a decision had been reached between the German Medical Director and me as to what hospital we would use in the event of a major trauma. Even though Dresden had a very good hospital, it was not fully equipped to handle major injuries. The Klinikum Berlin-Marzahn hospital in Berlin was the only reasonably close hospital capable of handling such an injury. It contained all of the ancillary services needed to deal with massive life-threatening injuries. These included a large blood bank, a vascular surgery team, intensive care physicians, and a full service laboratory. Even though the hospital in Dresden was only 10 minutes away, I knew Alex would die there. I was sending him to Berlin, 35 minutes away. I thought to myself; what if he doesn't make it to Berlin? I would be in deep shit! My decision to send him to Berlin would be second-guessed by physicians, nurses, family, and others forever.

In our rush to save Zanardi, Trammell and I had forgotten all about the other Alex. He arrived at the care center in a second ambulance just as we finished with Zanardi. Fortunately, Tag was fully awake and only complaining of back pain. Terry and I found nothing life-threatening as we examined him. He would need several X-rays after a shunt like that. Due to the extreme forces involved in such a high-velocity crash, we had learned to be concerned about subtle injuries not readily apparent on physical examination alone. We bundled him up for the second helicopter to Berlin. As we emerged from the med-center pushing Tagliani toward the second helicopter, we were appalled to see the chopper with Zanardi still sitting on the ground. I couldn't believe it! I ran to the door and grabbed the pilot by his shirt sleeve. Yanking him from the aircraft I pointed to the sky and yelled:

"Schnell, Schnell!"

He got the message! Pushing medics and onlookers out of the way, he prepared to lift off. By this time Daniela, Alex's cherished wife, had pushed her way past the security guards and was rushing toward her husband. Actress Ashley Judd, then fiancée of CART driver Dario Franchitti (they later married) and a close friend of the Zanardis, was with Daniela. I immediately jumped in front of them and told Ashley I didn't want Daniela to see her husband unconscious and without any legs. While I was discussing the situation with her, Daniela bolted for her husband. She reached his side and hugged him, whispering something in his ear. One of the helicopter crewmen later told me that Alex seemed to stir a little as his wife spoke to him. I realized I was wrong in trying to keep her away. Daniela's voice and her gentle touch clearly played a positive role in his battle to survive. At least he was still alive. I had grossly underestimated the strength and determination of a truly devoted wife.

The pilot hastily pushed Daniela aside and slammed the rear door of the helicopter. He shoved a medic, still fussing with the linens, inside and closed the side door. They finally left for Berlin. Probably six or seven minutes had been wasted on the ground fiddling with paperwork and protocol. I gave Alex less than a 50/50 chance to survive. My neck was stuck way out there.

Tag's helicopter followed closely behind Zanardi's. Chaos reigned on the helipad as more and more people arrived. Jon Potter came lumbering in along with Father Phil. I told Father Phil to go with Ashley and Daniela in a third helicopter. A fourth was arranged for Potter and Alex's attorney, they also took off for Berlin. It looked like a scene from the movie M.A.S.H. I ran back inside to contact the receiving hospital.

I called the emergency room physician and gave him a full report on Zanardi. I told him Alex would need to go to surgery immediately and not stop in their emergency room. Alex's injury was considered to be 100% fatal when it occurred in the field. No one, to our knowledge, had ever survived this injury for the simple reason that help couldn't arrive before the victim bled to death. Without proper medical care, death would usually occur in less than four minutes.

Terry and I had done everything we could. I went back into the medical center, plopped down in my chair by the phone, and waited. Terry went back to Safety 2 for the remainder of the race. There were still 13 laps to go. Neither of us gave Alex much of a chance.

While I sat there shaken and distraught, I wrestled with a thought that had repeatedly plagued me over the last 36 years. Why did I keep doing this? I had lost too many friends and consoled too many drivers and their families. I had been divorced twice and I didn't get to see my children and grandchildren often enough. I had very little free time and I was continually torn between two full-time jobs. When I wasn't at a race, I was managing the Neuroscience Intensive Care Unit at Jackson Memorial Hospital in Miami, Florida, the main teaching hospital for the University of Miami.

Why does anyone, for that matter, get so hooked on what is so often such a vicious and unforgiving sport? My mind drifted back to the beginning.

Chapter 1

THE RACE FAN
TURNS DOCTOR

A ll I remember is a red blur and a very loud noise. I was four when my parents first took me to the Indianapolis Motor Speedway. My father was a physician, off duty that day so it was probably a Wednesday. Most doctors in Indiana took Wednesday afternoons off in those days. We didn't stay long because I was soon crying from the noise. The impression made on me that day, however, was lasting. Now I'm 76 and still going to races. I didn't get to attend the actual race until I was 11, but I would listen religiously to the annual radio broadcast of the Indy 500 hosted by Sid Collins, the famous 'Voice of the 500'. He and his team of announcers actually made you feel as if you were in the cars. You could almost smell the hot rubber and oil as you listened.

The first race I attended was the Indy 500 in 1955. That race would also make a lasting impression on me. Bill Vukovich, my favorite driver at the time, was tragically incinerated in a flaming crash on the backstretch. I can still remember the thick black smoke rising, seemingly forever. The massive crowd of over 300,000 people grew strangely quiet as the race was halted. Tom Carnegie, the track announcer who is still there today by the way, eventually proclaimed that Vuky had been mortally wounded in the crash. I turned to my father and said cheerfully:

"Great Dad, he's just wounded!"

At 11 years old, I didn't understand the meaning of the word mortal. When my dad told me he was dead, I was devastated. But in spite of the loss of my racing hero, my passion for the sport continued to grow. Cutting classes in May became common all the way through college. In 1965, I graduated from Hanover College, a small private school located along the Ohio River in Southern Indiana. Following graduation, I was accepted to several prestigious medical schools. To my father's surprise, I picked Indiana University largely because it kept me in Indianapolis and close to the race track.

Soon after graduation, I married Emily Hyer, my high school sweetheart, and entered medical school that fall. The medical school campus was in downtown Indianapolis, less than five miles from the track. I convinced my new wife to move into an apartment on Georgetown Road, located just outside the fourth turn at the Speedway. We were mostly broke in those days, but happy. To me, the majestic grandstands that blocked our living room window made perfectly good scenery.

During my second year in medical school, an ad caught my attention on the bulletin board in the Student Union Building. It asked for volunteers to work at the Speedway. I hastily signed up and soon found myself inhaling the bizarre mixture of stale beer, mustard, and undercooked hotdogs that permeates the infield. I was initially assigned to a tent in the rain. There, I took care of mostly tired, drunk, but otherwise harmless people who were slogging their way through the mud-soaked infield that was Indy in May. This was the greatest automobile race in the world and I was now a part of it. Well sort of.

One day I asked my father how to get into the pits. He replied: "You have to know Joe."

I decided then and there to get to know Joe, whoever he was. The fact of the matter was you really did have to know Joe. Joe Cloutier was track owner Tony Hulman's chief operating officer. Tony owned the Speedway but Joe was the man in charge. When you met Tony, who had purchased the track from Captain Eddie Rickenbacker in 1945, he would smile, shake your hand, and greet you in his warm Hoosier way. Joe, on the other hand, rarely smiled. He would usually just sneer and glare at you as if your very existence was a matter of conjecture. Joe was Tony's hatchet man and most people around the Speedway were deathly afraid of him. For some reason, Joe took a liking to me and we remained good friends until his death in 1988. This friendship enabled me to have access to anywhere on the Speedway's grounds.

Dr. Thomas Hanna, the track's medical director, had always managed to stay on the good side of Joe while developing the track's infield medical center. He soon became my ticket to what I thought was the most hallowed ground on earth, the pits at the Indianapolis Motor Speedway. It didn't hurt that Dr. Hanna and my Dad were in the same bowling league.

I was asked to join the Speedway's medical staff that same year. I was ecstatic! By custom, you were not allowed to work at the track on the actual day of the race during your first year on staff. Raceday was only for the hardened veterans. This fact enabled me to go to the race as usual with my family. We sat in our reserved box in Grandstand 'E', the same seats we had been sitting in for over 20 years. Grandstand 'E' was in the first turn. My uncle had owned the seats since the early 40s. The year was 1965.

Near the end of the race, as I stood and watched excitedly, my new racing hero, A.J. Foyt, blew his engine while leading handily. Suddenly, from out of nowhere, I was hit on the head from behind with a full, unopened bottle of beer. The glass bottle exploded in a deluge of blood and suds into our box. Evidently, the well-dressed young man sitting behind me didn't like the fact that A.J. had retired either.

I was hit squarely on the right side of my head, lacerating my scalp. I was conscious after the assault, but bleeding profusely from a deep wound. My brother Tom, with help from one of my cousins, rushed me to the nearest first aid station located just beneath the grandstand. My face and scalp were caked with blood, so, by then, were my shoes and pants. The nurses gasped when I was ushered in and quickly hustled me into the nearby ambulance. Meanwhile, the jerk who threw the bottle had run from our box, but not before another cousin managed to grab his wristwatch. Luckily, it had his name engraved on it and we would find him later.

The ambulance took me to the infield care center. A small building located behind, and just south of, the garage area. Inside, a group of nurses and physicians from the local community were busily seeing other patients. It looked like a small town emergency room on the Fourth of July. The nurses placed me on a hospital bed where I met Dr. Zimmerman. Doc Zimmerman looked to be around 110 years old. He examined me and administered to my bleeding head.

"You're a lucky man", he said

Doc Zimmerman, it turned out, was an aging optometrist, not a real trauma guy, but he was Dr. Hanna's friend and therefore, he also knew Joe.

I survived the incident with only a bandaged head and a splitting headache for a reminder. The Speedway voluntarily compensated me for my ruined shoes and pants with a little extra cash for mental anguish. Their risk managers had learned long before to take an accident report on the spot. These kinds of incidents were not unusual at the Speedway and an early deposition, along with an offer to appease, saved the track a great deal of money. A couple of attorneys and a court recorder were on duty in the care center that day, a procedure that remains in place today.

I returned to the Speedway undaunted the following year, assigned to the care center for the month and in Heaven. Once assigned to the care center you could actually work on the race track. Sacred ground indeed! On a typical practice day Dr. Hanna would remain in his office in town while Doc Zimmerman manned the care center. The lowly medical student, me, would be assigned to the one and only ambulance stationed at the entrance to Turn 1.

Early in May of 1966, I found myself standing next to the shiny, red and white Conkle Funeral Home hearse. Their hearse doubled as the ambulance. It was stationed at pit out with a direct shot into Turn 1. There were no paramedics in those days so it was driven by the funeral home's embalmer. I waited anxiously for my first on-track rescue mission. There was nothing in the hearse except a bottle of oxygen.

I was only a second year medical student and knew virtually nothing about trauma care. No one else did either. Trauma protocols didn't exist in those days, and emergency medicine was not yet a specialty. The embalmer and I waited patiently.

Graham Hill, the 1962 World Champion, was in his 'rookie' year at the Speedway. Shortly after lunch, on that hot, steamy afternoon in May, the emergency horn located just behind our station shrieked loudly signaling a crash. I was standing just outside the ambulance enjoying the sun. When the horn shrieked, the embalmer and I both jumped. I was suddenly faced with a very difficult decision. Should I enter the back or the front of the ambulance?

While I was deciding which door to grab, the hearse/ambulance sped from the station. As it rushed by me, I hastily grabbed the rear door. Pressing the button on the handle, it luckily flew open. I held a death grip as the door swung me wide to the outside entering the first turn. As we approached the short stretch between Turns 1 and 2, the door slammed shut sweeping me inside. I was tossed, ragdoll-like, into the back of the vehicle. I cut both of my elbows on the stainless steel handrails as I tumbled past the gurney. I was then slammed heavily into the rear door as we accelerated through the second turn. We were gaining significant speed! The embalmer, a frustrated racecar driver, really loved doing this. He had the ambulance floored.

As a result of my indecision, I was again bleeding profusely at the Speedway for the second time in less than a year. We hurtled down the backstretch reaching speeds of well over 100 mph. When we reached Turn 3 we came to a grinding stop. The racecar we were chasing so aggressively had only spun harmlessly into the grass.

I was trembling all over, partly because of the wild ride in the ambulance, and partly because I was the medical officer in charge. At first, I wasn't sure what to do. I managed to regain some of my lost composure as I ran up to the driver who was sitting quietly in his now motionless racecar. Oh God, it was Graham Hill! With voice quivering, I shouted down to him:

"Are you OK?"

He calmly looked me in the eye, slowly folded his hands carefully beneath his chin, and, with his signature mustache quivering said in his classic British accent:

"I'm fine, but you look bloody awful!"

With horror, I realized I was bleeding substantially all over his brand new Dunlop driver's suit.

It was common practice in those days for race tracks to contract with funeral homes to provide their ambulance service. Regular ambulance services were few and basically confined to the city's streets. Gallows humor in Indy was; if the hearse turns left leaving the track it was going to Methodist Hospital and the driver might live, if it turned right it was going to Conkle Funeral Home and the driver was dead. In the 60s one out of seven drivers died in the major forms of auto racing including Formula One, so a right turn was not that uncommon.

Dr. Hanna ran a 'tight ship' in the infield care center. The system he had developed was, without question, the best and only true medical system dedicated to the safety and wellbeing of racing drivers anywhere in the world. It was manned by a group of dedicated nurses, most from nearby Methodist Hospital, who worked tirelessly in the care center alongside a volunteer staff of over 20 physicians. During the 11 months of the year that the famous race track sat idle, Dr. Hanna practiced as a family doctor in a small office in Speedway, Indiana, less than a mile from the track. What he knew about trauma care he had learned by the seat of his pants. He rarely worked on the race track, preferring to remain in the care center where he found himself on the receiving end of some of the worst trauma imaginable. Drivers Eddie Sachs, Dave MacDonald, Bill Vukovich, Jim Malloy, Pat O'Connor, and Art Pollard were just a few of those killed on the track. In those days, there was little anyone could do to save a badly injured driver.

Sachs, MacDonald, and Vukovich were all killed instantly in fiery crashes. Pollard, a close friend of Dr. Hanna's, died of a broken neck and head injuries on the first day of qualifying in 1973. When a driver did manage to make it to the care center alive, he would be seen and initially treated by Hanna. He invented motorsports medicine as far as I am concerned, and I am forever indebted to him for getting me started at the 'Greatest Spectacle in Racing'.

I graduated successfully from medical school in 1969. My wife and I still lived off the fourth turn at the Speedway, and by this time so did several of the Indy 500 drivers. To me this was truly life in the fast lane. I met Johnny Rutherford and his wife Betty while living on Georgetown Road, as well as driver Carl Williams and racing artist Ron Burton. A.J. Foyt would often visit a special friend of his who lived there, so I got to meet him as well. When I wasn't working at Methodist, I would hang out in the apartment complex and listen to the drivers lie to each other. Eventually, I got to know some of them quite well and on occasion would even get to accompany Williams to one of the local race tracks in order to test his sprint car. With the engine in the front, a sprint car isn't as fast as an Indy car but they carry 900 horsepower and on a half-mile track are a major challenge to drive – even to the most skilled veteran. They were raced aggressively on short tracks scattered primarily throughout the Midwest, and the East and West coasts.

During the fall of 1969, we took Carl's sprinter to an open test at Winchester Speedway in Winchester, Indiana. An open test is where a group of car owners rent a track for the day to test and develop new ideas to make their cars go faster. The drivers like them because they're a chance to gain valuable track time. As was customary in those days, there was no ambulance in attendance. Open tests were considered very dangerous. At least 20 cars were scheduled to practice at racing speeds.

Winchester Speedway is a steeply banked, half-mile paved oval with a reputation for being treacherous. I was the only medical person in attendance, and I was just an intern! Early that afternoon Bruce Walkup, a very aggressive but not exceptionally talented sprint car driver, suddenly lost control of his racecar. He bounced violently, end-over-end down the front straightaway. I watched the whole crash from the pits, about 40 feet away. Bruce came to rest directly across from where I was standing. I ran to the car to help pull him out. He was 'dingy', having no idea what his name was, what he had been doing, or where he had come from. He complained of severe neck pain. Stabilizing the neck of an individual after a big crash was just coming into vogue. Being a modern and up to date young physician, I attempted to do this with the only thing I could find, a folded up, dirty bath towel. We had been using the towel to wipe the car off each time it came into the pits. Terrific neck support! With no ambulance there was no backboard. Most ambulances back then didn't carry them anyway.

Steve Stapp, Williams' car owner, helped me lay the injured Walkup on an old wooden door recently removed from an adjacent building. We then stuck him into the back of Stapp's Chevy station wagon. A former racer himself, Stapp drove like a madman to the Winchester Hospital, about 12 miles away.

We came to a screeching halt in the driveway of the tiny little emergency room. Carrying Walkup on the door, we rushed inside. Once inside, we found ourselves immersed in a dark void. It was pitch black. No one was home. In 1969, 24-hour emergency room care was non-existent in big cities let alone small towns. I went berserk, a common occurrence when frustrated in those days, and yelled frantically into the abyss. No response.

I felt along the walls and managed to find a light switch. I flicked it on. Just as I did, I was confronted by a huge, take-up-the-whole-hallway kind of small town nurse.

"Who the hell are you?" she asked.

"I'm Dr. Olvey", and I need X-ray and a neurosurgeon, stat!" Stat meant immediately.

She laughed out loud and asked us all to leave. As she whirled around to head for the exit, she added angrily:

"The surgeon's on the golf course, and I'm not about to call him for any stupid race driver!"

She hurriedly left the room.

Staring at each other in disbelief, we gathered up our patient and headed out the door. Back into the station wagon and on to Methodist, a real hospital. The attitude of the nurse was not uncommon in those days. Drivers were considered by many to be brave, but dumb. If they were injured, they deserved it. No one looked at automobile racing as a real sport, but more as a daring act of thrill seeking.

Indianapolis was about 70 miles away. Luckily, Walkup appeared to have sustained only a minor concussion. He woke up in the car after having lapsed into unconsciousness for a short time in the little emergency room. He was still complaining of severe neck pain. His main injury seemed to be a muscle and ligament strain to his neck. But I was just an intern.

We sped into the parking lot outside of the Methodist Emergency Room and rushed Walkup inside. He spent a couple of hours getting X-rays and a proper examination by a neurosurgeon. He was soon released after everything turned out fine. The next morning he called me complaining loudly of what we affectionately called racer's rheumatism. He found it very hard to get out of bed the next morning because he was sore all over.

Walkup was able to race the following Sunday at Winchester, although still in a lot of pain. Unlike many of today's stars, drivers in those days would tolerate a lot of pain just to be in a racecar. Many of the drivers' sole source of income was what they made in prize money. Dick Simon, in fact, once drove the entire Michigan 500 with most of the bones in his right wrist broken. Al Unser Sr. drove a race at Mid-Ohio with a temperature of more than 103 degrees. And Troy Ruttman managed to finish the Indy 500 one-handed in 1952 after his right arm had been severely burned during a pit stop.

Drivers in the 60s frequently raced or tested without qualified medical personnel in attendance. No one knows how many fractures went untreated, simply allowed to heal on their own. Concussion likewise often went undiagnosed. Duane Carter Sr., father of Indy 500 veteran Pancho Carter, told me about a weekend of sprint and midget car racing that was probably not unique in those days. He crashed heavily one Friday night in a sprint car race. He knew this because of the newspaper clippings his wife showed him the following week. As the story goes, he groggily refused to go to the hospital after the crash and had his wife drive him to another track for a midget race the following night. He competed in a third race on Sunday afternoon. On Monday, he discovered three trophies sitting on the breakfast room table but had no recollection of having received any of them.

The number of drivers who raced immediately after a significant concussion is probably staggering. One has to wonder how many accidents may have occurred or how many injuries or deaths resulted because a driver continued to race after a minor injury to his brain.

Deaths in Indycar racing continued to plague the sport throughout the early 70s. The danger from fire, once a leading killer, had lessened considerably after the use of gasoline was banned in 1965 following the fiery deaths of Eddie Sachs and Dave MacDonald in the Indy 500 the year before. The hideous crash had turned many fans against the sport. Head injury then stood alone as the number one killer of racecar drivers, and remains so to this day.

A race driver was actually considered fortunate after a big crash if he sustained only a concussion. Most head injuries during the 60s and 70s were severe and frequently fatal. Little protection was available for the driver's head. Helmets lacked full face coverage and had little in the way of inside padding. The cockpit was made of bare aluminum with the sides cut low, almost completely exposing the driver's torso. This design offered virtually no protection from flying car parts and other debris. Repeated concussions were common, and several drivers should probably have retired earlier than they did. Among the drivers that died during this period was young David 'Swede' Savage. Savage did not die of a head injury or burns, as was reported. His death was the result of a colossal medical screw up.

Savage crashed violently in the oft rain-delayed race of 1973. It resembled a plane crash more than it did a car wreck. When the smoke settled, only his seat, still burning with him in it, remained on the race track. The rest of the car was completely torn apart and scattered throughout the exit of Turn Four. Remarkably, he was still conscious when rescuers arrived. Reportedly he told the rescue squad:

"Holy shit, I've sure made a mess of things haven't I?"

Savage spent the next 31 days in the Intensive Care Unit at Methodist Hospital. I was his resident physician at the time. Savage required a ventilator to support his breathing due to severely bruised lungs and was on the kidney machine due to renal failure. In spite of all this paraphernalia, he was still able to joke with the nursing staff. One morning he went so far as to fake a cardio-respiratory arrest, much to the chagrin of his nurse. His positive attitude was remarkable in spite of his severe burns and multiple fractures. I was optimistic that he would eventually survive the crash in spite of his many injuries.

Suddenly, for no apparent reason, his liver failed acutely. He died shortly thereafter from fulminate hepatitis. His liver had been totally destroyed, the result of live Hepatitis B virus particles being injected into his bloodstream from a bottle of contaminated plasma. The plasma was part of a tainted batch inadvertently distributed throughout the United States. Several other unfortunate people died in hospitals around the country. The inevitable class action suit soon followed.

Savage had always been a free spirit, a charismatic new breed of driver. Instantly popular with the fans, he was handsome, funny, and talented in many areas. One of the first drivers to come into the United States Automobile Club from sports cars, he was a tremendous loss to the racing world. Too many drivers like Savage had died both in Europe and in the United States as a result of racing accidents. The danger of the sport was becoming intolerable. Incidents in Europe had not only killed several drivers, but many spectators as well. In 1955, during the famed 24 Hours of Le Mans, a Mercedes racecar driven by Pierre Levegh crashed into a crowded grandstand, burst into flames, and killed more than 81 spectators.

Politicians from around the world began to demand that the sport be banned. These demands, usually arising after a series of fatal crashes, were growing more numerous. To this day motor racing is not allowed in Switzerland. The acceptance level for death in all sports was changing worldwide. Spectators were no longer willing to tolerate death on such a large scale. Safety in motorsports was fast becoming a major issue.

Chapter 2

USAC TAKES
A FIRST STEP

Life on the Championship Trail, as the United States Auto Club Indy car series was named in the early 70s, was a constant challenge to driver safety. Track medical directors were often poorly qualified, or totally inappropriate for the job at hand. Often close friends of the promoter, they were basically race fans who got free passes to a race, but had no idea how to handle a true emergency.

Hearses, usually advertising the name of a local funeral home, doubled as ambulances as at Indianapolis, and were primarily for transportation since they rarely contained any rescue equipment. Most race tracks did not have an infield care center. When they did, it was often ill equipped for any serious medical care. Treatment tables were frequently adorned with brownies, ham, coleslaw and other delicacies for lunch, making their use in an emergency nearly impossible. Nurses were often there primarily to socialize, harboring lusty thoughts of snagging a famous race driver for a long-term relationship. Dealing with a real emergency was not on the agenda. Get the injured driver in the ambulance and get him out of here, was the order of the day.

At the famous old Milwaukee Mile, the first permanent race track ever to stage an Indycar race, the hired physician was an elderly obstetrician. He wore a full-length white lab coat on the race track when attending a crash and bore a striking resemblance to Ichabod Crane, the tall skinny character in *The Legend of Sleepy Hollow*. At the high banked, very fast track in Atlanta the medic was an aging, retired eye doctor. At Pocono, there was no doctor in attendance at all, and the ambulance was not even a hearse. It was an old station wagon driven recklessly around the grounds by the track's caretaker, who had no medical credentials whatsoever. Helicopters, when you could get them, were usually of the morning traffic variety, not really suitable for transporting an injured patient. The Indianapolis Motor Speedway for years was the only race track with a proper emergency medical system. Promoters at other tracks meant well, but organized and proper medical care was expensive and therefore scarce.

In addition to poor medical care, the drivers had to contend with poor protection in their cockpits. Helmets, until the 60s, were flimsy compared to today's models with no standards for testing their integrity. Very early helmets were made of leather and did no more than keep the driver's hair out of his eyes. Metal replaced leather in the 40s, offering some protection from flying bits of debris. Fiberglass did not become available until the 60s, with greater development in the 70s to include an energy-absorbing inner liner. Having the liner in place resulted in a marked improvement in mortality from traumatic brain injury. Helmet standards were developed in 1973 in the US, somewhat earlier in England.

Fire-resistant clothing didn't make an entrance until the 60s, and even then it was often shunned by the drivers. Bobby Marshman, a great driver on short ovals, was burned to death in 1964 while testing a car at Phoenix International Raceway. He was wearing only a pair of jeans and a cotton tee shirt. It was hot that day and he felt it would be more comfortable in jeans than in the firesuits of the day.

Seatbelts were not made mandatory until 1963. Drivers until then were convinced they were better off being thrown clear of a crash rather than risk being trapped in the car and burned alive. During the era of the tubular framed front-engine cars, being ejected was often the best option. As long as you weren't run over by another competitor or thrown into a solid object like a tree or the wall, you were less likely to be hurt than if you remained strapped in the car. In those days, most of a crash's energy was transmitted through the tubular frame directly to the driver in the cockpit. Wrecked cars during the 60s would often look fairly good after a crash that killed the driver. They could frequently be repaired by the next weekend following the death of one driver, allowing a new, and up and coming driver, his chance to compete for fame and fortune.

Shoulder harnesses, although available, were frequently not used. Drivers who did use them would often wear the belts too loose to do any good. Worn in this fashion, drivers could be semi-ejected during a flip, risking severe neck and head injuries as their torsos were abruptly held in check by the belts, allowing their heads to continue accelerating.

Seats, in those days, were simple aluminum structures without good support or padding. Rarely, a driver would even sit on the bare floor of the car using cushions or pillows as padding. As a consequence, drivers were often tossed about like dolls, suffering many secondary injuries inside the cockpit during a crash. Drivers and officials alike wanted desperately to improve the safety of racecars, but there was virtually no scientific data available to guide any rule changes. Design changes were usually made on hunches and gut feelings of the crew members. Drivers, being very superstitious by nature, were reluctant to make changes of any kind. They were painfully slow in accepting new ideas. Public outcry, and worry within the sport itself, did eventually lead to some much needed mandatory changes in the mid-70s.

Seatbelts and shoulder harnesses were finally mandated along with fire-resistant uniforms. Colin Chapman, designer of the famous Lotus racing cars and a true engineering genius, designed the first monocoque chassis. The engine, gearbox, and suspension all bolted on to this new chassis design. The driver now had a safety cell or tub in which to sit. The tub was surrounded by energy-absorbing, breakaway components that would dissipate much of the kinetic energy associated with a crash. When one of these new rear-engine cars crashed, it would explode in a spectacular display of fragments, often allowing the driver to walk away unscathed.

Unfortunately, some racing organizations still fail to adopt many of these safety regulations and continue to allow racing cars that are undesirable from a safety standpoint. For example, some racing cars still use tubular frame technology with little in the way of energy-absorbing capabilities. Until only recently, one major racing organization left safety issues up to the driver and his team. The reason given was that they didn't want the liability associated with rule mandates. This attitude is unlike the majority of major series. One well-known stock car driver once told me that he could race in a tee-shirt and flip flops if he wanted to. Tragically, there have been a number of injuries and some deaths over the years due to the use of antiquated designs, and a reluctance of some sanctioning bodies to mandate safety improvements readily adopted by other organizations.

During the Milwaukee Indycar race in 1974, Gordon Johncock, a driver who truly believed the shortest distance between two points was a straight line regardless of the track's configuration, crashed and badly fractured one of his legs. The track's safety crew arrived quickly, extricated him, and loaded him into the waiting ambulance. The ambulance attendants – there were only a few paramedic rescue units in service throughout the entire United States in 1974 – hurriedly prepared to leave the scene. Unfortunately, in their haste, they failed to lock the patient bed, or gurney as it is called, in place, and also failed to latch the rear door. As a result, Johncock slid unceremoniously from the back of the ambulance as if being buried at sea. He tumbled to the pavement in agony and, as the story goes, refused to get back in:

"I'm better off in my racecar than I am in that fucking thing," bellowed the 1973 Indy 500 winner.

Wally Dallenbach, a good friend of Johncock's and a fellow driver at the time, observed the entire fiasco. This most recent debacle was the culmination of a series of dangerous mishaps that had occurred during on-track rescues that season. It was the proverbial straw that broke the camel's back. Dallenbach was incensed with the variability of on-track medical care and ambulance services in the 70s. Track safety depended on what state the race was being run in, who provided the ambulances, and how honest and caring the promoter was.

Dallenbach approached Dick King immediately after the Milwaukee race. King was president of USAC at the time and very much wanted to improve the safety of the sport. King himself ran a funeral home and ambulance service. Dallenbach had been harboring an idea for some time and suggested a traveling medical team to King. He was the first driver or other participant to do so. Ironically, the Formula One Grand Prix circuit was considering the same option in Europe for the very same reasons. Medical care in Europe was much the same as in the United States, with a lot of variability between countries. Led by reigning World Champion, Jackie Stewart, the Grand Prix drivers were demanding improved and consistent medical care at their various tracks.

King contacted my office to arrange a lunch meeting. Dr. Hanna had just appointed me Assistant Medical Director at the Indianapolis Motor Speedway and as such I was the logical candidate to put such a team together. King and I met at the Speedway Motel in the winter of 1975. He asked me if I knew any doctors who would be willing to go to the races, not get paid, risk their lives, ruin their marriages, and perhaps lose their jobs for the sake of the sport. I thought about it for around two seconds and hastily replied:

"I would!"

He asked when I could start and I told him I could be ready by the next race. Obviously, I could not do all of the races by myself and still remain in the fulltime practice of critical care medicine. I would need some help. I was fortunately able to enlist the services of another young physician and racing enthusiast by the name of Dr. David Clutter. He took nearly as long as I did to accept the offer. I had met Clutter while working at the Speedway a couple of years earlier. He too had signed up at the University to work at the track during the month of May and we were in competition for

Dr. Hanna's attention. In addition to Clutter, I added my resident at the time, Bruce White. White was soon graduating from the surgery program at Methodist and he too was a big race fan. White was developing into a damn good surgeon and he admired the seemingly carefree spirit of the drivers. Clutter and White both jumped at the chance. The USAC medical team was born, the first of its kind in the world!

Dr. Hanna soon named Clutter the other Assistant Medical Director at the Speedway. Our competition for the good doctor's attention grew daily. Clutter also loved fast sports cars. Sadly, he lost his life one beautiful spring morning in 1976 while driving on 16th street in Indianapolis *en route* to the Speedway. A huge garbage truck, driven by an idiot, ran him off the road and into a ditch. The truck landed on top of Clutter's brand-new Datsun 240Z, crushing them both. Clutter died instantly from the massive injuries sustained in the crash. He was a promising young physician and a real loss to the city of Indianapolis and to the sport of automobile racing.

Following Clutter's death I invited Dr. Henry Bock to join the team. Hank, as he was called, was another race fan who became a doctor. I knew him from both Methodist Hospital and the University. I had a great deal of respect for his abilities as a physician, and he was a fun person to be around. He also took Clutter's place at the Speedway as one of Dr. Hanna's assistants. Bock entered his medical career as one of the first emergency room physicians in the state of Indiana. The specialty was new and he was on the ground floor. He was, and still is, dedicated to saving lives and has always been politically correct.

A bachelor, Hank in those days surrounded himself with beautiful women. He is still at the Speedway as its Medical Director, and is also Director of Medical Services for the Indy Racing League. He remains actively involved in research for injury prevention while still providing hands-on care at the race track. He has markedly advanced the medical system Dr. Hanna put in place at the Indianapolis Speedway into what is now one of the most sophisticated of its kind in the world. Similar systems have been put in place in other parts of the world, such as Silverstone in England, and the Paul Ricard facility in France. Spectators at Indianapolis have expert medical care virtually at their fingertips. If you're going to have a heart attack, you are likely better off having it during the 500 Mile race than in your own home.

White was the original 'Alfie'. He was handsome, charismatic, and full of ideas on how best to enjoy life. He spent a number of months with me as my resident taking care of patients in the intensive care unit. More than just another resident, Bruce and I became good friends. Off duty we would talk mainly about racing and girls. I was divorced at the time and with my good friend's help I started dating, something I hadn't done for over 18 years.

In 1976, I was living the single life high atop the Summit House, an apartment building located near downtown Indianapolis, only a couple of miles from Methodist Hospital. In a weak moment, Bruce and I decided to have a party in May to celebrate the race and we invited everyone we knew. We didn't know for sure if anyone would show up, but we were going to have one hell of a party. Indianapolis was very busy in May and it was only four days until the race when we made this decision. There were a lot of other parties for people to go to besides ours, so we honestly didn't think we'd have many guests. Surprisingly, nearly everyone we invited showed up. Linda Vaughn, Miss Hurst Golden Shifter, was there with A.J. Foyt. Fellow drivers Johnny Rutherford, Parnelli Jones, Pancho Carter and Johnny Parsons Jr. also came. Actor James Garner, safety guru Bill Simpson, and international businessman Teddy Yip were there. Radio announcer Paul Page, newspaper columnist Robin Miller, Lieutenant Governor Larry Conrad, track announcer Lou Palmer and several other drivers and racing celebrities came as well. Unfortunately, so did the police! Some of the residents, it seemed, had complained about the noise. Our guests, being politically very powerful, convinced the police politely to inform the residents to live with it and go back to sleep. The race in May was indeed a very big deal!

In the spring of 1978, Bruce was assigned to cover the April USAC race in Trenton, New Jersey since I had to be on call at Methodist Hospital and was unable to attend. To his surprise and delight, he was invited to go to the race with the top USAC officials in a chartered twin-engine plane owned by a hotshot local pilot. He called me the day before he was to leave, very excited to be traveling with the 'big guys'. They left for the race on Thursday in the unpredictable weather that characterizes the Midwestern part of the United States in the spring.

When he arrived in Trenton, Bruce called me stating that he didn't much care for the pilot. According to Bruce, the guy kept looking back at the passengers talking to them about racing instead of flying the plane. I told him if he was that uncomfortable, not to fly back with them. He could easily find a ride back to Indy with someone who had driven to the race. He laughed, said he was on call the next day, and told me not to worry.

Dr. White died that night along with five other top USAC officials. The plane, a non-pressurized turboprop, nose-dived into a cornfield after losing direction and stability in a violent thunderstorm over eastern Indiana. It was estimated the plane hit the ground at over 400 mph. Commercial flights in the area at the time had all diverted to alternate airports because of the storm. Not this guy.

The crash made a huge hole in the ground several feet deep. Identifying the bodies was nearly impossible. The pilot had once bragged to a group of people in the bar at the Speedway Motel about how he had managed to land a plane once during a violent hailstorm with no windshield. The National Transportation and Safety Board, not surprisingly, ruled that pilot error was the cause of the crash.

The police asked me to help identify Bruce's body the following morning, or at least his personal effects. Fortunately, they were able to make the identity using dental records and I didn't have to go to the morgue. I'm not sure I could have done it. I took Bruce's death very hard. I had never lost a close friend before. Now I was the only USAC doctor left of the original three. Pretty scary!

A combined funeral was held for the victims of the crash at the Episcopal Church on North Meridian Street in Indy. The service was attended by nearly everyone who had anything to do with Indycar racing. USAC had to reorganize and so did our shattered medical team. Dr. Bock and I carried on, although we were both gravely saddened by the deaths of Clutter and White. I never took life for granted again.

Chapter 3

CARTER CRASHES
AT PHOENIX

Pancho Carter, arguably one of the best sprint car drivers of all time, was testing a car at Phoenix International Raceway in the fall of 1977. Phoenix, like a lot of tracks in those days, made extensive use of steel barriers. Wooden poles, widely separated from each other, supported the twin steel rails of the barrier. A gap of at least four inches separated the two strips of railing. Track management had other priorities so they had not replaced the rapidly aging barriers. Many of the wooden support posts were rotting and the metal rails were bent and twisted from earlier impacts. Corporate suites and other sponsor amenities held a higher priority with the promoters, as they often did. Concrete is expensive and promoters would habitually cut corners on safety unless they were forced into submission by a strong sanctioning body, an outraged media, or governmental regulations.

Carter lost control of his car late in the day, and drove nose-first into the inside barrier along the front straightaway. He was traveling in excess of 160 mph. The nose of the car penetrated the two steel rails midway between two of the wooden support posts. Grinding between the sharp-edged rails, he was abruptly stopped when he met one of the wooden posts broadside. Nearly decapitated from the initial impact, he was slammed into the heavy post at the level of his pelvis. He was critically injured as a result of the crash. His wife Carla, sitting on the scoring stand, was forced to witness the entire incident.

I was at home eating dinner in Indianapolis when I received the urgent call from her. She told me that there had been a horrible crash and her husband was headed to Good Samaritan Hospital by ambulance. She was afraid he was dying. The hospital was in downtown Phoenix, about 30 minutes away. He was bleeding severely when they removed him from the car and he looked to her to be in a state of shock. Tubs were aluminum then and easily distorted, offering little in the way of side impact protection. I told Carla I would contact the trauma center immediately. I also told her that Pancho was very strong and if anyone could survive such a crash it was him. There was nothing else I could do.

After several tries, I finally got through to Good Samaritan; the news was not good. Carter had sustained a badly fractured pelvis with the broken bones crushing his right sciatic nerve, the big nerve that controls movement in the legs. He had lost a large amount of blood due to the pelvic fractures and had also ruptured his bladder. The doctor told me over the phone that Carter would never drive again and would be lucky ever to walk again. Carter was the reigning champion of both the USAC Sprint and Midget car series and had also been named Rookie of the Year at Indianapolis in 1974. Most of us in racing felt that he was destined to be the next A.J. Foyt.

His recovery in Phoenix was agonizingly slow. The course his doctors had charted aimed for a slow rehabilitation with a sedentary, non-athletic lifestyle the ultimate goal. Few physicians in those days paid much attention to athletes, let alone racecar drivers and their desire to get back into competition. The prevailing medical opinion was they were lucky to be alive and should take up something else for a hobby or pastime. Sports were not looked upon as real jobs by many physicians. Carter refused to accept this approach, and so did I. I advised him to sign out of the hospital against medical advice and come back to Indianapolis. He did this without hesitation. When I met him at the airport, I thought I might have made a terrible mistake! He was thin, gaunt, and weak as a kitten. He couldn't walk. He looked pathetic sitting in his wheelchair. He in no way resembled the athlete he was before the crash.

I admitted him to Methodist Hospital, where he began a very intensive rehabilitation program. The goal was to enable him to drive again as soon as possible. The rehabilitation specialists in Indianapolis were accustomed to dealing with race drivers and treated them as the highly skilled athletes they were. Race drivers are generally dedicated, focused, and above all want to race again no matter what hardship might lie in their way. I've seen drivers who had to practically crawl or even be carried to their cars in order to compete. My policy has always been to allow a driver to race if he or she has the desire and they can safely demonstrate good control of the car without putting themselves, or anyone else, in unnecessary danger.

Carter worked hard. Three months after his crash, unable to lift his right foot due to the severe nerve damage, he won his first race back in competition. His victory occurred on the tough, five-eighths mile oval at Indianapolis Raceway Park located just six miles from the famed Indianapolis Speedway. Limping to his car at the start of the race, he didn't look like a contender at all. He was wearing a brace fitted to his right foot. The brace allowed him to work the throttle in and out using his thigh muscles, instead of up and down using his ankle. It was the first appliance I can remember that was made specifically for a driver to allow him back into competition. Carter was back in business!

Once he got seated in the car, he became the same old Pancho. A fierce competitor, he won his comeback race going away. He would go on to win many more, as well as the Sprint car title again. He would also do well in Indycars, where he could run competitively with anyone on an oval track. Road courses would always be a problem for him, however, due to the severe nerve injury and his inability to move his foot from throttle to brake quickly enough to be competitive. This handicap would eventually lead to his retirement as more and more road races were destined for the Indycar schedule. The horrible crash in Phoenix was the beginning of the end of a very promising career.

The doctors there told him as he left against their advice that he would never be able to drive a passenger car again, let alone race. He and I greatly enjoyed sending them the newspaper clippings of that big win at IRP!

Carter's story was one of many that involved racing drivers and their remarkable recoveries following severe, career-threatening injuries. I have often been asked if I thought race drivers were superhuman. The answer is no, they are not superhuman, they are driven. They are compulsive competitors and will try to beat each other at anything whether it's racing cars or doing push ups. Like the tough farmers of Indiana, their level of compliance with doctor's orders is nearly perfect. All they want to do is race. I have never once had a driver tell me he wanted to retire because of an injury. They all ask, as soon as they are able to talk:

"Hey doc, when will I be able to get back in the car? "

Chapter 4

CART

In 1978 a group of prominent car owners, encouraged by former Formula One and Indycar star Dan Gurney's so-called 'white paper,' became disgruntled with the way USAC and the Indianapolis Motor Speedway were managing the racing series. The group felt strongly that they were not sharing a big enough piece of the pie. They argued that the purse at Indianapolis, even though large, did not conform to the percentages given the teams at other races. They were concerned that USAC raced over and over in the same tired venues without giving much thought to expanding the sport into other parts of the country, to include road racing and eventually international events.

Led by car owners Pat Patrick and Roger Penske, a meeting was held in Indianapolis to form a new organization. This new body would be charged with sanctioning all future Indycar races with the exception of the Indianapolis 500. The 500 would continue as a USAC-sanctioned event. The goal of the new organization was to broaden the scope and appeal of American open-wheel racing as well as to increase the bottom lines of the owners. The sport had truly become stagnant! Several tracks, like Trenton, Phoenix, and Milwaukee, had two races per year while other parts of the country had none. USAC had become a 'good ol' boy' organization with little forward thinking. The new organization was to be named Championship Auto Racing Teams, or CART. Unlike NASCAR and Formula One, each of the owners would have an equal voice in the operations. This new series would be owned and managed solely by the owners.

The Speedway and USAC didn't think too highly of this group of revolutionaries and promptly filed a lawsuit to ban the original six owners from competing in the 1979 Indy 500. A bitter court battle ensued that the Speedway lost, basically because they were in violation of the right to work laws. The owners blacklisted at Indy included Patrick and Penske, Gurney, McLaren team principals Teddy Mayer and Tyler Alexander, oilman Jim Hall, and real estate and tire magnate Bob Fletcher.

The court battle left in its wake many hard feelings among the USAC stalwarts. These feelings remain largely unresolved to the present day. John Frasco, CART's lawyer who won the case, would later become one of CART's many CEOs. Under his leadership, CART would become a major force in international motorsports, eventually developing a large television audience, sell-out events, and a dedicated fan base.

Shortly after the formation of CART, I received a phone call from Mr. Patrick, who asked me to join the new organization as their Medical Director. He told me that CART placed safety as a high priority and they wanted to duplicate the Safety Team that we had put in place in USAC. As an enticement to change sides, he offered me a small stipend to attend the races. USAC, at the time, was paying only my expenses. To his surprise, I promptly said no. Even with the incentive, out of loyalty to USAC and the friends I had made there, I elected to remain with the Speedway and their established series.

The next phone call I received, not more than an hour later, was from none other than A.J. Foyt, who was still my racing hero.

"Hey, Olvey! Fuck those guys in USAC. CART's the way to go!"

This was magic, because A.J. was like a God to me. As far as I was concerned, he could do no wrong. I promptly said yes, and in so doing burned all of my carefully built bridges at the Speedway. Bock remained with USAC and assumed my role as medical director. A.J., in true Foyt fashion, went back to USAC in less than a week, following a heated argument with Pat Patrick, Roger Penske, and the rest of the CART owners. Foyt would go on to vacillate between the two series for the next several years.

I needed another partner after Bruce White's death so I asked a cardiovascular surgeon friend of mine if he would like to share the CART duties with me. Dr. Harold Halbrook was not a major race fan, but he loved the glamour associated with racing. Dealing with open heart surgery on a daily basis made him more than suitable to handle any emergency that might arise. Halbrook agreed to work a few of the races, but not without some trepidation. He didn't last long and soon decided to resign.

After Halbrook resigned, I hired another resident of mine, Dr. David Crippen. Crippen was fanatical about critical care and had recently finished a fellowship in that specialty. The sicker the patient, the better he liked it. He developed into a unique physician. Before entering medical school, he served with the special forces in Vietnam. He often found himself in the thick of the fighting and was shot down over the jungle on four occasions. As a result of his heroism, he was awarded the Bronze Star. He would later suffer from night terrors and flashbacks, especially while sleeping in motel rooms. Crippen had no fear, however, a big asset on the race track and when caring for the critically ill. In later years, he would climb Mount Everest without oxygen, race motorcycles, and continued to fly support in medical helicopters long after most doctors had given it up.

He eventually left Indianapolis for Pittsburgh, where he became a professor and an expert in critical care and the management of pain and sedation. Unfortunately, routine ailments take up at least 90% of a physician's time. As a consequence, Crippen was not the most tactful physician in practice and his bedside manner left a little bit to be desired unless you were really sick. He would easily become bored with the mundane and we all sensed it. Those of us on the Safety Team likened him to the 'jaws of life' extrication tools. He was not afraid to tackle anything in the field and was a hit with local emergency crews. Time constraints would eventually require him to give up the CART series.

About this same time another character was emerging at the

Speedway as well as within CART. His name was Jon Potter. Potter grew up in Indianapolis, graduated from high school in Warren Township, and became a deputy sheriff in Marion County. When not busting heads as a policeman, he led a country rock band as a diversion and had performed on occasion at the Grand Ole' Opry.

I first met Potter at a New Year's Eve party in the old, and very traditional, Indianapolis Athletic Club. Jon was fortunate to be born with the gift of perfect pitch and taught himself to play both the piano and guitar at an early age. This particular New Year's Eve he and his band were the entertainment in the club's posh third floor ballroom. Potter could play the piano just like, and as good as, Jerry Lee Lewis; at the time my favorite country entertainer.

Potter had been asked by the club's management earlier in the day to give the folks in the audience a night they would always remember. Always willing to please, Potter had a plan. At the end of his show, he began to play Jerry Lee's 'Great Balls of Fire'. Partygoers, well lubricated by then, began dancing wildly on the tables, throwing things, and generally acting crazy. Midway through the song, Potter pulled a can of lighter fluid out of his jacket pocket and soaked the keys of the piano. He then produced a lighter and set the piano on fire without missing a single beat of the song. The Steinway baby grand burst into a wall of flames! Smoke filled the ballroom! Alarms sounded, and several people ran panic-stricken into the cold January air. Many of us were too drunk to go any place so we stayed and enjoyed the bedlam. It was a night to remember, no question!

I had to meet this guy! I stumbled up to introduce myself while the maintenance men extinguished what was left of the blaze. Potter and I hit it off right away. We soon discovered our mutual loves; Jerry Lee Lewis and Indycar racing. We became close friends. Potter had been a race fan for as long as I had, developing an interest while in grade school. His favorite driver at the time was Bobby Unser. He had also developed a close relationship with the Hulman family, mainly through his work as a deputy sheriff. He would cleverly garner duty at the Speedway during the month of May and was slowly getting to know everyone involved in the 500, especially Joe Cloutier and Tony's daughter Mary.

The following April, Unser approached me at the spring race in Phoenix. Bobby wanted to know what I thought of Potter and would he be a good executive director for the new drivers' organization being proposed. The Championship Drivers Association, as it would be called, was planned primarily to benefit those drivers who could not fully support themselves. The CDA would help drivers find sponsorship, get disability insurance, and work out reasonable travel arrangements. Most drivers in those days did not make the big salaries that many of them do today and younger drivers needed a lot of direction to get started. The new organization would also provide a much-needed voice for the drivers when dealing with their owners who pulled all the strings.

I told Unser that I had only recently met Potter and I didn't know much about his character, but he sure played one hell of a piano! Soon thereafter, Potter was named the organization's Executive Director. The original idea for the CDA had also come from Wally Dallenbach.

The Indycar drivers, through their voice in the CDA, were able to push for safety improvements at the tracks they race on as well as in the cars they drive. A benevolent fund was also created that benefited a number of deserving individuals and charitable organizations through the years. Potter also established the CDA's 'CARE' program. When a driver crashed and was taken to the hospital, Potter, or his designated representative, would also go to the hospital to handle the driver's entourage, deal with the media, and act as the surrogate when no family member was present. This was a major comfort to the drivers and their families.

CART's medical program was rapidly expanding during this period. They had a Safety Team like USAC, a traveling physician to provide continuity at the varying venues, and they had the CDA to provide supportive care to the drivers and their families. They also had a Safety Director.

Steve Edwards was another character in the growing mix of

personalities. Like me, Edwards transferred to the CART series from USAC. He and I had worked together in USAC for almost three years. When USAC president Dick King first told Edwards that I was joining his Safety Team, he wasn't thrilled. In fact, he was fairly angry. He didn't see how a doctor was going to help any on-track emergency situations. He was certain I would just be in the way and would likely get run over. He didn't realize that, unlike most other physicians of the day, I was enamored with critical care and learning all I could about emergency life-saving procedures. Like emergency room doctors, critical care doctors were a new breed of physician in the 70s.

When I first came on board with USAC, Edwards was highly suspect and remained somewhat distant from me. After three or four races, however, he warmed up a degree, recognizing the fact that the doctor was there to stay. We soon worked reasonably well together and developed a satisfactory division of labor. I was glad to be with him in CART and the organization welcomed us both with open arms.

Accustomed to being in charge at the scene, Edwards wanted everything to be a certain way, his. When not attending a race, he worked professionally as one of the first paramedics on the streets of Tampa, Florida. He continued to have some reservations about physicians being allowed to roam freely on his race track, but generally tolerated me. Long before I had joined USAC, Edwards had been their Safety Director, and as such, had been unchallenged. He seemed to think of himself as a race driver, albeit without a car, and lived vicariously through his Safety Team.

Edwards lived and breathed racing safety, so much so that he tended to neglect other things in his life. His dedication consumed him to the point that he would occasionally appear to complicate incidents on the race track so he, and only he, could straighten them out. He would occasionally put himself in harm's way, just managing a narrow escape as the wheels of a speeding racecar tattooed his fire-resistant uniform.

Occasionally, he would manage to put those of us seated in the truck with him in some jeopardy. We never actually crashed, but we had some close calls. Once, in Long Beach, we were on our way to a crash speeding over the long, gently curved section of Shoreline Drive that made up the front straightaway. Edwards enjoyed using the racing line whenever he could, so he was running about five feet from the outer wall, drifting gradually toward it at close to 100 mph. I was seated next to him in the passenger seat as usual, tightly gripping the door handle.

From out of nowhere, Al Unser Sr. popped into my side view mirror. Edwards, focused on his driving, didn't see him at all. Unser was closing fast! He was committed to his line, not expecting a safety truck to be lumbering along in front of him. It was too late to alter course! Just when I thought we were all going to die, Unser miraculously squeezed his racecar into the small space separating our truck from the retaining wall. Small bits of debris shot up from between our truck and the wheels of Unser's speeding racecar. It was that close! The instant we were passed, you could not have jammed a piece of cardboard between our truck and his car. Needless to say, Big Al was not real happy with the Safety Team that day.

The concept of the Safety Truck originated with Edwards in USAC. The trucks were designed as rapid response vehicles carrying everything needed to effect a safe extrication of an injured race driver. By putting everything we needed into our two trucks, we were able to keep the number of on-track rescue vehicles to a minimum. We carried emergency resuscitation equipment, splinting material, dressings, extrication tools, oil dry, and, very importantly, a big fire extinguishing apparatus.

A huge fire boss adorned the back of the truck with the capability of fighting a very large fire. Several small handheld extinguishers were also readily available for smaller blazes. Indycars burned methanol and water was the best material to extinguish the blaze. Using chemicals other than water could damage engine components, only stifle the fire, and potentially turn the whole scene into a slippery mess.

The idea was to arrive at the scene of a crash as quickly as possible, extinguish any fire, and then attend to the injured driver. Once the driver was safely out of the car, the scene would be restored to its pre-crash configuration with the track cleaned of any and all debris. The Safety Director acted as foreman, directing all operations. The two firemen with us on the crew took care of the fires and handled the complex and heavy 'jaws of life'. The physician was in charge of the driver's resuscitation and also assessed the scene for injuries to officials, spectators, or crew members depending on the location of the crash.

In the beginning, CART could afford only two Safety Trucks to provide rescue and clean-up at the events. We named them CART 1 and CART 2. Eight races were sanctioned during CART's first year. The entire series was organized out of Pat Patrick's headquarters in Jackson, Michigan. We carried a traveling crew of only eight officials and four of them were assigned to the Safety Team.

The original team included Steve Edwards, as director and the only paramedic, Neal Carter, a retired midget and sprint car driver as general helper and fireman, Skip Richmond, one of Neal's old mechanics, and me. Steve and I rode in CART 1 while Neal and Skip manned CART 2. With only four men working on the race track, we were easily overwhelmed. As a consequence, we became multi-talented. It was not unusual to see the doctor sweeping up oil dry or doing the famous oil dry two-step. This dance is an unusual gyration resembling a form of jitterbug that forces kitty litter or similar substance into spilled oil to absorb it following a crash or a blown engine.

The four of us once worked an entire 500 mile race at the now defunct Ontario Motor Speedway in California, with a full field of 33 racecars. We were spread pretty thin that day but managed to work a number of crashes and to keep the event moving. We were young and foolish, except for Neal, and didn't mind the fact that we were nearly run over on occasion.

One of these occasions occurred on a sticky, miserable summer day at Mid-Ohio, a track located in the middle of nowhere between

Columbus and Cleveland. A storm had been brewing during the late afternoon practice session. When the storm finally broke, sheets of rain pummeled the track. Visibility went to zero and the ground actually shook in response to deafening claps of thunder. Lightning bolts pierced the black sky as if we were under some type of aerial attack and the wind bent some of the trees nearly 90 degrees.

During the height of the storm lightning struck one of the corner stations, knocking all four of the workers to the ground. The heat and electricity badly singed a couple of them. The four resigned their post en masse, running rapidly toward the parking lot. Edwards and I, being the only ones in the vicinity, were forced to cover the badly damaged station as the racecars groped their way back to the pits.

We abandoned our truck and took over the station's mangled communication equipment. While we were assessing the damage and organizing the remains of what was left of the station, Joe Saldana, a mediocre driver in the series, spun wildly off course. Why he was going that fast on his way back to the pits in a driving rainstorm is anybody's guess.

He slid sideways on the wet grass, seeming to pick up speed as he went. Clods of mud and dirty water were violently tossed in our direction. We promptly bailed out of the soggy station, leaping to the side as Joe continued unabated. He finally crashed heavily into an adjacent tire barrier, flipping over in the process. He came to rest upside down at a 45-degree angle with the tires.

When Edwards and I approached the wrecked car, Saldana was pinned against the tire wall with only his helmet visible as it dangled between the inverted car and the wet grass. It was still pouring down. After regaining our composure, we cut his belts and eased him out of the car. He was badly shaken but awake and alert. Another near miss!

Following this particular incident, safety barriers, lacking before, were strategically placed around all corner stations to protect the exposed workers. Prior to Saldana's crash, corner workers were left on their own to escape a crashing racecar or flying piece of debris. Bravery is one thing, being stupid is quite another. It always amazed me as to the number of volunteers the tracks could find who were willing to expose themselves to errant, speeding racecars with no barrier protection at all.

We were soon able to add two new firemen and another paramedic to the original Safety Team. Dave Crippen and I continued to alternate races providing the physician coverage, while Neal Carter and Skip Richmond did most of the dirty work. The two new firemen resembled longshoremen more than they did firefighters. They were big, tough guys, Greg Passauer and Dave Hollander. Passauer was a good old boy from West Hickory, Pennsylvania and Hollander was a heavyweight out of New Jersey. Hollander joined CART fulltime after helping us on a number of occasions at our Pocono, Pennsylvania events. He was strong and gruff on the surface, but had a softer side of respect and loyalty for the organization and the people in it. Passauer was your basic mountain man with a heart of gold that was as big as he was. Hollander and Passauer were both certified firemen. The new paramedic was Jerry Guise from Indianapolis. I had worked with Guise in Indy during the month of May. He was well versed in extrication and life support and a welcome addition to the team.

Life on the road was spartan, but we were all thrilled to be an integral part of the events. Try as we might though, we could not get the brass in CART to allow Port-O-Lets, the little green or blue outhouses, on, or even close to, our safety stations. Consequently, we soon developed enormous bladder control. We were, in fact, not regularly supplied with the little houses until one of us was caught live, on television, pissing on a fire truck at the famed Michigan International Speedway. The track in Michigan was then owned by millionaire businessman, Roger Penske, a stickler for detail. Penske didn't think that outhouses added to the grand looks of his race track on national TV so they had been outlawed. The risk of one of us caught on TV was worse, however, so Penske finally allowed the relief stations in discreet locations.

Sitting in the Safety Trucks was not glamorous. We would often spend 10 to 12 hours straight on some lonely corner in 90-degree heat. We were not allowed to run the air conditioner for fear of spilling water on to the race track, or overheating our engine. No one thought to bring us water in those days so we were in a state of continuous dehydration. With the windows down, bees and wasps were also a constant threat. Telling exaggerated stories about our personal lives and past adventures became the order of the day. We rapidly became a fairly tight-knit group, a sort of one for all, all for one arrangement, and none of us would trade it for the world!

Chapter 5

FOYT HAS TROUBLE
IN DAYTONA

Threatening them at times, A.J. Foyt remained loyal to USAC through 1981. He returned to the CART series in 1982, mad at USAC for something only he understood. I'm convinced that he missed the competition afforded by the likes of Mario Andretti, Al and Bobby Unser, Johnny Rutherford, Gordon Johncock, Wally Dallenbach, and a host of others. He and I continued our friendship as though he had never left. In February of 1978, he asked me to go with him to Daytona for the famous 500. He agreed to pay my expenses and guaranteed we would have a good time.

I was ecstatic. I had never been to that part of Florida and had only seen the big NASCAR race on closed circuit TV. A.J. had heard horror stories about the medical care provided at the track from some of the other drivers. He wanted his own physician to be there in case anything bad happened to him during the race.

I flew to Daytona and met A.J. and his crew at the Hilton Hotel on the beach. Because of job commitments, I couldn't leave Indy until the weekend so I didn't arrive in Daytona until early Saturday afternoon. The big race was the next day. The rest of the team had been in town for five or six days and was already acclimated. A.J. had qualified well for the race and was one of the favorites to win. He was in an unusually good mood when I arrived. He and the crew invited me to dinner that night at a cowboy bar located near the race track. We spent the evening listening to A.J. tell hilarious stories from his past.

He talked about the time he tried out his newly purchased, large-caliber machine gun behind his Houston auto dealership. In the potentially hazardous incident, he attempted to fire the huge gun like Arnold Schwarzenegger did in *The Terminator*. Unleashing a stream of deadly bullets, the force of the powerful gun knocked him to the ground. After losing control of the weapon, he managed to inflict significant damage to an adjacent office building as the bullets marched progressively up the concrete and windowed exterior. Luckily, no one was injured.

In another story, he described how every morning, on his way to his car dealership, he would be met at the only traffic signal *en route* by a young man in a heavily modified coupé of some kind. The kid's car had every aftermarket go-fast device available. When the light turned green he would blast off, leaving Foyt sitting angrily at the intersection. Growing tired of this daily embarrassment, A.J. and his crew worked all night to install one of his stock car engines in the pick-up. The next morning he rumbled up to the stoplight with flames popping out of both exhausts, and waited for the kid. The kid turned up as expected. When the light turned green, this time the kid found himself totally engulfed in noxious blue tire smoke. A.J. never saw him again. Story followed story and we didn't leave the bar until late in the evening. The big race was early the next morning.

Wanting to please A.J. and leave no stone unturned, I awoke very early and headed straight to the track. I arrived in the team's pit area before any of the crew. On the way, I had stopped briefly at a 7-Eleven convenience store to purchase a large styrofoam cooler, some sports drinks, water, and ice. I also bought several bottles of soda; the kind A.J. liked. The weather forecast was for a hot and muggy day and I wanted to prevent any potential heat-related problems with the team.

I packed the big green cooler full with ice and drinks and set it discretely in the rear of the pit, out of everyone's way. When finished, I had nothing else to do so I just sat down on the pit wall and absorbed the early raceday morning ambiance of Daytona International Speedway.

A.J. and the crew arrived soon after I had finished packing the cooler. He was walking toward me from the garage area flashing that famous grin of his. I was still sitting on the wall gazing at the vast horde of good ole' boys and southern speed freaks. As A.J. approached, he couldn't help but catch a glimpse of the bright green cooler out of the corner of his eye. He came totally unglued! He grabbed a tire iron and, as his face turned a deep purple, he smashed the cooler to smithereens. Again and again, he pummeled the hapless cooler until there was nothing left and cans were scattered everywhere.

"What muthafucka put this here!" he yelled. "I'll kill the sumbitch!"

I tried desperately to become invisible. I remained motionless and quiet. A.J. continued his tirade for a good 15 minutes. He kicked at various objects and widely scattered some of the pit equipment before slowly regaining his composure. He stomped off to get dressed for the race.

It started with no one the wiser. Green, it seemed, was still taboo with many of the old guard in racing. At least, it was with A.J. I didn't think it mattered so much any more since Jimmy Clark had won Indy in a green car way back in 1965. Live and learn. I sure hoped it didn't bring the team any bad luck.

On lap 68 A.J., while leading the race, suddenly lost control of his car entering Turn One. I watched horrified as he spun wildly in front of me. He flipped upside down, and then rolled side-over-side six or seven times before coming to rest in the grass. The ambulance seemed to take a long time to get there. There was a ridiculous rule at the time that didn't allow any rescue vehicles on to the racing surface until the full field of cars had passed the start/finish line. This delay, on a long track, could be extensive and quite serious when a driver was on fire, in a coma, or bleeding heavily.

The ambulance and firecrews eventually arrived at the scene and pulled him unconscious from his wrecked car. He was taken to the infield care center where the track doctors decided they had better fly him to the hospital downtown. I sank to a new low...

Michigan millionaire and true gentleman Jim Gilmore, A.J.'s car owner at the time, grabbed me hurriedly and we jumped into the rental car. We headed downtown to Halifax Hospital. When we arrived in the emergency room, no one was there except for a couple of big old nurses. Shades of Winchester Hospital with Bruce Walkup! I demanded to see a doctor.

"They're all on the golf course or at the race," said a seemingly put-out nurse.

I couldn't believe it. Gilmore, by this time, had located the hospital administrator on call and told him to get down to the emergency room as soon as possible. When the administrator arrived, we calmly informed the poor guy that Jim McKay and ABC's entire *Wide World of Sports* entourage was *en route* for live interviews. He promptly gave me full staff privileges and placed Gilmore in complete control of the hospital's communication system.

"We don't need this," I think he said.

I proceeded to examine A.J. who was slowly coming out of his coma. A radiologist thankfully arrived and agreed to accept my orders for X-rays and a CT scan of the brain. I admitted A.J. to their observation floor to await the neurosurgeon. His condition was stable and he had regained consciousness. As he sheepishly looked up at me his first remarks were:

"Hey doc, I'm getting too old for this shit!"

A.J., of course continued to race for many more years, repeating the same comment to me years later when he crashed badly at Elkhart Lake, Wisconsin in 1990. Knowing he was going to be OK, I headed back to the track to do an interview with Formula One champion Jackie Stewart, then color commentator for ABC's broadcast. By now it was pitch dark and everyone had pretty much left the facility. The program's producer decided the best place for the interview was on the roof of the main grandstand. He felt the roof location would present a more dramatic backdrop for the unfolding story. This *was* the legendary A.J. Foyt, and calls were pouring in from all over the world.

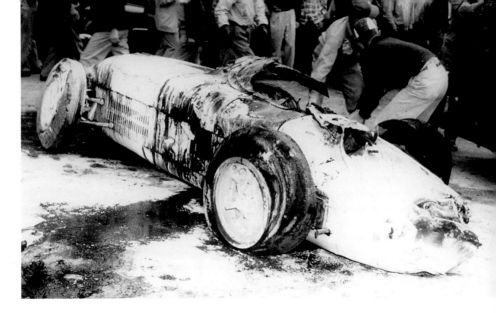

ABOVE *The aftermath of Bill Vukovich's fatal crash at the Indy 500 in 1955. In those days, drivers often fared worse than the car.* (Author)

RIGHT *Colin Chapman with Jim Clark at Indy in 1963 with the Lotus 29. Chapman had a brilliant mind, Clark was a brilliant driver. They succeeded with the rear-engined monocoque chassis first introduced to the United States by Jack Brabham and Cooper in 1961.* (Motorsport Images)

BELOW *Pictured here is the 1958 version of the Conkle Funeral Home ambulance. In 1966 the location, set-up and the anticipation were the same.* (Indianapolis Motor Speedway)

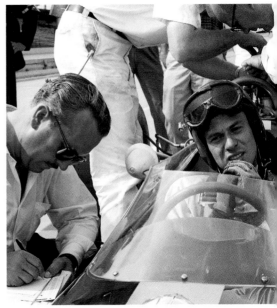

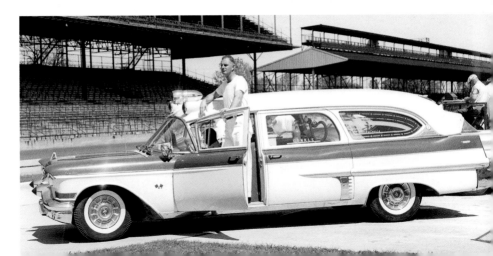

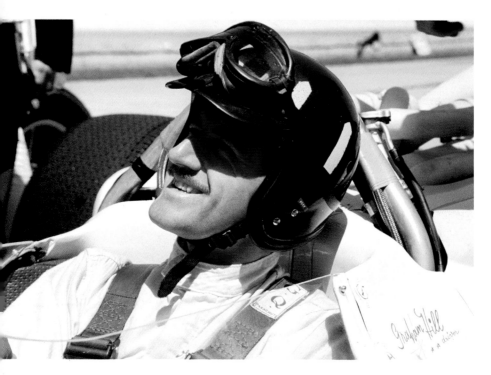

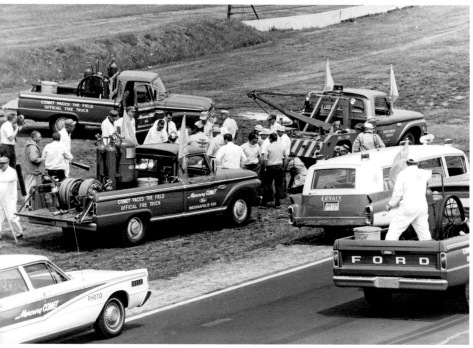

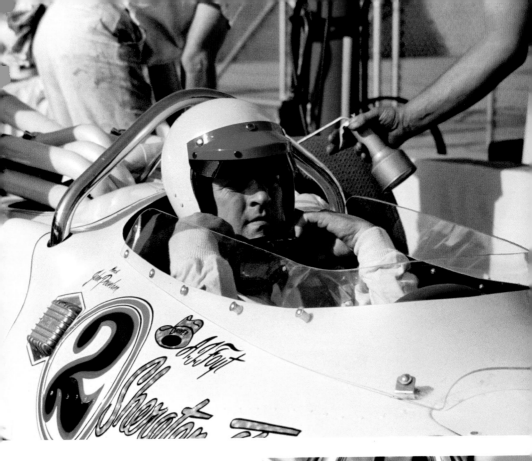

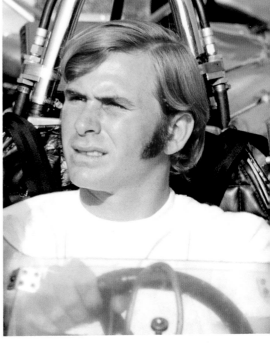

Opposite top *Graham Hill preparing for the 1966 Indy 500, which he went on to win. Same look he gave the author.* (Motorsport Images)

Opposite bottom *The Conkle ambulance/hearse on the scene of what is thought to be Graham Hill's spin in 1966.* (Indianapolis Motor Speedway)

Above *A.J. Foyt at Indy in 1966. Tough on any track and a hero to many, A.J. survived racing's most dangerous years.* (Motorsport Images)

Right *'Swede' Savage brought the Californian movie-star image to open-wheel racing, as well as great talent. He died way too soon, at the age of 26.* (Motorsport Images)

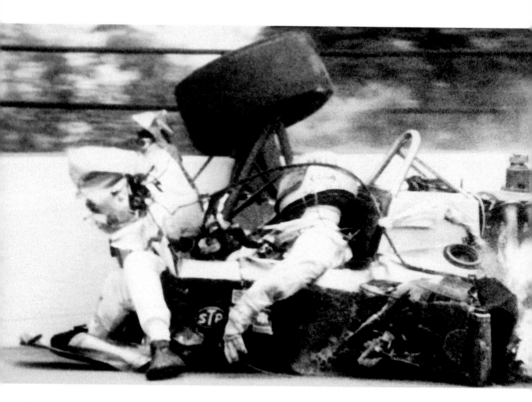

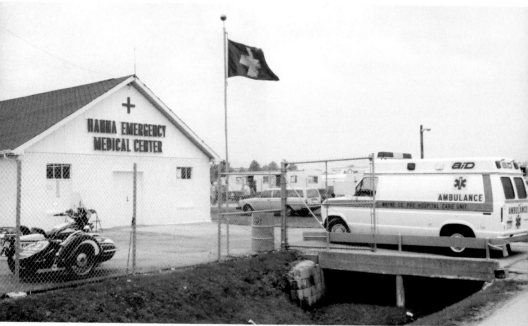

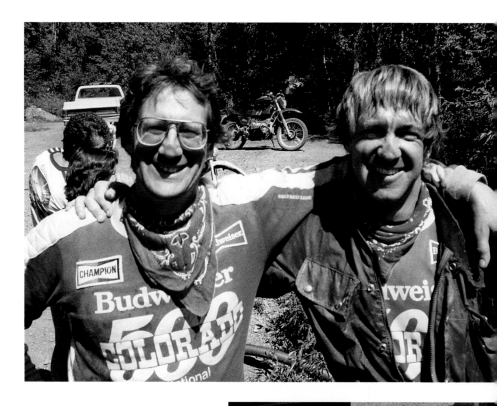

OPPOSITE TOP *Danny Ongais' Interscope racecar comes to rest after his accident at Indy in 1982. If you look closely, you will see the hole through which part of his leg went over the wall.* (Author)

OPPOSITE BOTTOM *1982, the year Danny Ongais crashed at the Speedway. The Medical Center, now named for medical pioneer Dr. Tom Hanna, takes in another injured driver.* (Indianapolis Motor Speedway)

ABOVE *Dr. David Crippen with the author after a hard day on 'The Ride' in 1982.* (Author)

RIGHT *Sir Jack Brabham and the big boss of 'The Ride', Wally Dallenbach.* (Author)

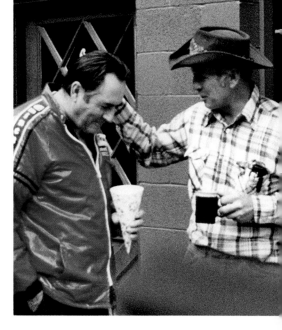

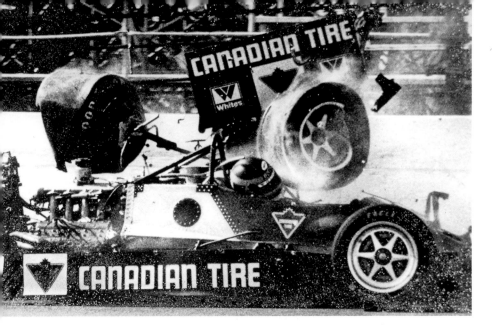

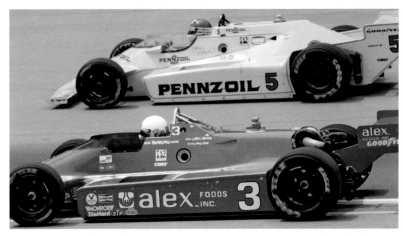

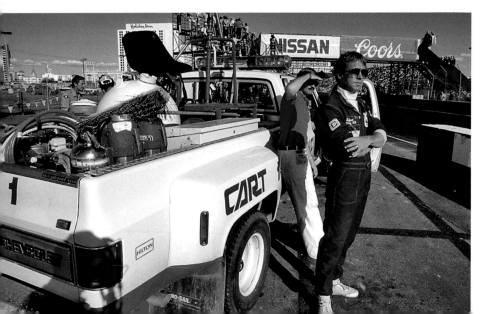

OPPOSITE TOP *Gilles Villeneuve's brother, Jacques, suffers a severe concussion at Indy as his exposed head is subjected to errant debris in the new carbon fiber tub.* (Author)

OPPOSITE CENTRE *Pancho Carter and Johnny Rutherford at speed at Indy in 1982.* (Motorsport Images)

OPPOSITE BOTTOM *The author contemplates the day ahead next to one of the original CART Safety Trucks.* (Dan R. Boyd)

RIGHT *Danny Sullivan walks the pits at Indy while his Penske team-mate, Rick Mears, uses his scooter to ease the pain upon his return to racing after his crash at Sanair in 1984.* (Dan R. Boyd)

BELOW *Rick Mears and 'The Magician', Dr. Terry Trammell, chat at pit side.* (Dan R. Boyd)

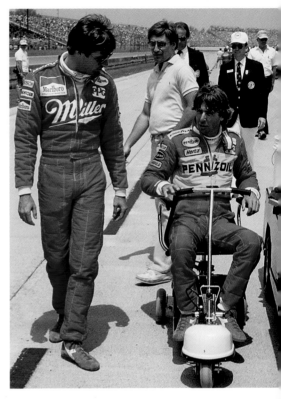

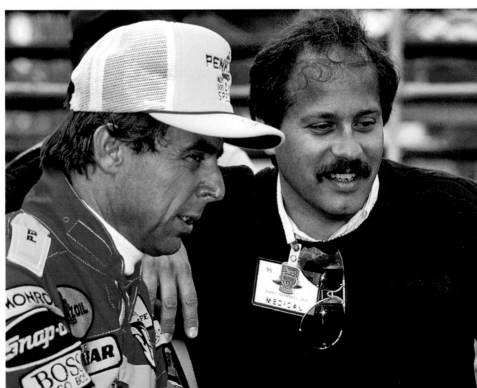

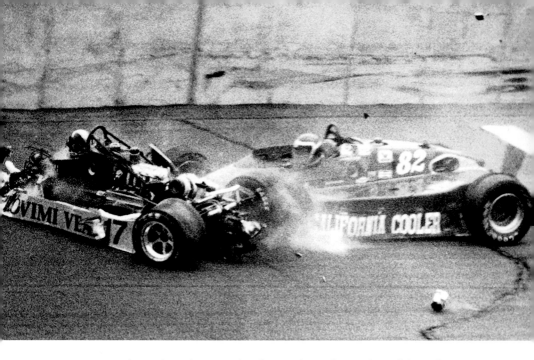

ABOVE *John Paul Jr. T-bones Derek Daly at Michigan, keeping him off the wall and inadvertently saving his life.* (Author)

BELOW *Daly comes to a stop. Extrication was easy, with the entire front of the car torn away by the crash.* (Author)

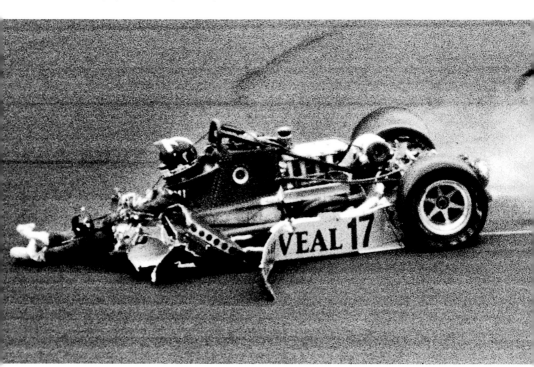

I had never done a live interview before so, for the second time that day, I was petrified! Stewart was real easy to work with and the interview came across well. I left for Indy the next morning after A.J. was released from the hospital. He never found out about the green cooler. I wrote a scathing letter to the CEO of Halifax Hospital as soon as I got home. I let him know what I thought about the fact that no one was on duty in his emergency room, the day of one of the biggest sporting events in the country and in full view of the entire world. The events of the day had made me keenly aware of the vast difference in the safety provided by NASCAR and the safety provided in USAC and CART.

Chapter 6

RUTHERFORD
DOES PHOENIX

Phoenix International Raceway was always one of my favorite tracks. Located in a picturesque setting west of the downtown, it was right on the edge of the Pima Indian Reservation, the area where our government decided to confine this particular tribe. CART had chosen Phoenix for its first race back in 1979. When we first started racing there, the sky was clear and you could see forever. Over the years that changed. By the late 80s a brown haze had enveloped the city thanks to smog from Los Angeles and the millions of cars driven by the people who had moved to Phoenix during the 60s and 70s hoping to improve their allergies.

PIR was a tough track. Shaped somewhat like a 'D', there was a big dogleg going down the backstretch. The turns were banked enough that if the car was set up right you could take them almost wide open. As a result, there were many big crashes there. The races were hotly contested, however, and the danger was tolerated. Johnny Rutherford liked Phoenix, too. In 1980 he was racing the famous Chaparral 2K racecar run by Texas oil millionaire, and former driver, Jim Hall. He was in command of the race like he had been earlier that season in winning his third Indy 500.

It was Death Valley hot on raceday with a track temperature of over 140 degrees. Steve Edwards and I were stationed in CART 1, located as usual between Turns 1 and 2. We were wishing the race were over so we could get out of our steamy firesuits and get something cold to drink. It was the last race of the season and we were ready to party. Suddenly, the all too familiar call came over the radio:

"Yellow, yellow, yellow, crash on the main straightaway."

We left our station spewing sand and gravel into the blue Arizona sky. As we came smokin' out of Turn 4, we watched helplessly as Rutherford's pit crew rushed on to the track and gathered around JR's bright yellow upside-down car. Meaning well, they hurriedly flipped it right side up. Rutherford landed with a bang as the car fell back on to all four tires. I shuddered as I watched his unsupported head and neck flop loosely side to side.

"Hope he's not paralyzed!" I yelled to Edwards.

We arrived at the scene fighting our way through scores of well-meaning crewmen, media, and other officials who had escaped from the pits. Somewhere in the huddled masses was JR. This is what always happened when someone crashed directly in front of the pits. Edwards and I charged into the fray.

When I finally reached the car, I found the biggest paramedic I had ever seen straddling the cockpit with both hands on Johnny's shoulders yelling at him:

"Look at me and no one else! Pay attention to me only! Ignore all these other people!"

Great, I thought, just what I needed to make my day. I politely asked for the medic's attention and was completely ignored. Unable to get anywhere near Johnny I retreated, enlisting the help of two, just as big, Arizona deputies. I told them to remove the paramedic who was now beginning to undress Johnny and do vital signs on him as he sat in the steaming car. Remember, the track temperature was over 140 degrees and we were standing in direct sunlight.

One of the reasons to have a physician who knows racing injuries on the race track is to be able to cut certain corners in order to effect a more direct and appropriate level of care. In this instance, Rutherford was restrained in an oven, unable to escape on his own. He had a good pulse, but was somewhat confused. There was no airway compromise, and he was not bleeding externally. The more time it took to get him out of the car the greater danger he was in due to dehydration and potential heat stroke. The paramedic was doing exactly as his protocols said. His protocols, however, were for a field situation where there is no direct medical control, not a hot race track with a competent physician in attendance.

My two deputies grabbed the medic, lifting him off the car. They hauled him through the massive throng into the infield. I don't know what happened to him after that. I informed another medic in attendance that if I could feel the pulse in Johnny's wrist then his blood pressure was adequate, at least for the time being. Johnny was beginning to come around and I thought it best to get him out of the heat as rapidly as possible. He was soaking wet, drenched with the sweat of more than two hours of racing in the heat of the day.

We stabilized his neck and placed him in the waiting ambulance. The damage, if any, had already been done when they flipped the car over. Luckily, JR was moving all four of his extremities by this time so at least he wasn't paralyzed. From the ambulance, he went into the helicopter and on to the hospital in downtown Phoenix; about a 15-minute flight. I went in the chopper with him along with his wife Betty, a former nurse from Indianapolis. The two of them had met in the mid-60s when he crashed practicing for the Indy 500. Rutherford was dazed and confused, but making some sense by the time we reached the emergency room.

He was admitted overnight with a minor concussion. He was lucky to have survived the crash as well as his flip right side up, not to mention the aggressive, misguided paramedic who would have him die of heat stroke. I made a note to myself that we needed a rule to keep everyone in the pits and off the race track in the event of a crash on the main straightaway, no matter what the circumstances.

With the system we had in place, expert help would arrive at a crash in usually less than 30 seconds. The rule was made, but the problem of interference by well-meaning individuals would continue to raise its ugly head over the next several years. I reported happily on Johnny's favorable condition at the end-of-the-season banquet held that same night and left for home the next morning.

Chapter 7

CART Ventures Out
of the Country

In October of 1980 CART would venture outside the United States for the first time. A race was scheduled in Mexico City. Many of us in CART had never been outside the United States and the trip to Mexico promised adventure. In fact, less than 10% of the American public even had a passport. By that time, I was married to my second wife, Diane, and we had become good friends with Al Unser Sr. and his wife Karen. The four of us traveled to Mexico together on American Airlines out of Dallas.

The night we arrived a big party had been arranged at the home of Josele Garza, a dashing and charismatic young Mexican driver whose family was very rich. Diane and I went to the party with Al and Karen by taxi. No one in their right mind would think of driving a rental car in Mexico City. As we pulled up to the enormous Garza house, situated high above the smog-laden city, we were flabbergasted. Al casually remarked that behind the big wooden entrance doors there would likely be security guards armed with large-caliber machine guns, waiting to interrogate us.

Sure enough, as the massive doors opened we were approached by a group of Che Guevara lookalikes holding weapons larger than they were. Leather belts adorned with bullets crisscrossed their chests. Fortunately, the guards turned out to be friendly and we enjoyed the party immensely, getting back to the hotel sometime early the next morning.

After only three hours of sleep, I went to the race track with Dr. Crippen who had flown in the night before. There was a lot of work still needing to be done if there was going to be a race that weekend. Crippen and I joined Steve Edwards and the rest of the Safety Team already at work inspecting and cleaning the track. The racing surface was filthy, with all matter of debris strewn about. We found everything from babies' pacifiers to prophylactics. In addition to the filth, several of the retaining walls were bare, exposed to the elements without the impact protection afforded by proper tire barriers. Tires in Mexico, it turned out, were hard to come by as most of them were being used on some sort of vehicle.

While we were busy sweeping the track, a large, mangy looking dog suddenly bolted on to the race course. He was one of many we had seen roaming freely around the city. Some, it appeared, had previously been skinned and were hanging up for sale at several roadside stands. The dog was obviously frightened and was making a real nuisance of itself. Security around the track was tight. About every hundred feet or so there was a Mexican policeman armed with an automatic rifle. These cops had been put there to keep out bandits and other freeloaders who might break into the facility. One of the cops, after watching the hapless dog for awhile, approached me calmly and asked if the dog was a bother. I said that he was. The cop replied:

"No problemo signor."

The next thing I remember is hearing several deafening bangs fired off in rapid succession, followed by the sight of the poor dog flipping end-over-end to its death 50 feet away. Things were certainly different in Mexico.

The track was ready for competition by the next morning and we all arrived very early. I was standing in the paddock, about 30 feet from the Penske transporter, waiting for the first practice period to start. Suddenly, I was overwhelmed with a sensation of extreme vertigo and what I thought were visual hallucinations. It occurred to me that I might actually be having a stroke. Panicked, I looked up to see a very tall TV tower writhing like a cobra in front of me, its guy wires undulating violently. When I dropped my head to look at the track, the pavement appeared to be unfurling before me, waving like a large black flag in a stiff breeze. Then it dawned on me, this was an earthquake!

The tremor lasted for about 90 seconds, long for an earthquake. When it was over, I found myself standing right up against Penske's transporter. It, or I, had somehow moved 30 feet during the incident. Everyone in the paddock was scurrying around yelling or pointing this way or that. No real damage had been done, but it took several minutes for everyone to relax.

We soon regained our collective composure and the day continued without incident. Bobby Unser took pole position for the race the next day. When we returned to our hotel that evening we learned that the quake had been a big one. Two people had died in Mexico City proper, together with several others close to the epicenter 80 miles away. The hotel across the street from ours lay in rubble. Thankfully, ours was still standing but everything in our room was topsy-turvy. Mexico was indeed becoming quite an adventure.

The night of the quake Diane and I decided to go out for dinner with the Unsers and Al's car owner, Bobby Hillin, another big oil man from Texas and relatively new to auto racing. We were riding to the restaurant in a large taxi on an always-busy Mexican thoroughfare. We soon found ourselves stuck in an enormous traffic jam. We were stopped just before an overpass and could see traffic streaming endlessly in both directions on the road above.

In Mexico, there were three different bus fares. One fare allowed you to ride inside the bus, another allowed you to sit on top of the bus, and a third let you hang on the side of it. Waiting patiently for the traffic to clear, we observed a bus chock-full of passengers lumbering slowly on the road above. All three fares had obviously been sold out. As it drew even with us, one of the passengers sitting on the roof slid helplessly off the back of the bus. He fell hard to the pavement below. Immediately, he was run over by at least 10 cars. Looking like a stuffed doll someone had tossed from an airplane, he was trampled repeatedly by the oncoming traffic. He had be on the pavement for a while, then in the air for a while, then back on the pavement. The poor man finally came to rest, dead, at the edge of the road. No one stopped! No one even slowed down! The traffic finally cleared and we continued to the restaurant. We were speechless. Mexico was truly different.

Raceday broke sunny and warm. Sunny in Mexico means that the sun was barely visible through the smog-browned haze, but you could tell it was there. With five minutes left before the start, the promised medical helicopter was nowhere to be found. I continually asked the local promoter where it was and I was continually told it would be there before the start. I realized deep down that there would be no helicopter. I hastily prepared an alternative plan. If we had a badly injured driver, we would use Penske's helicopter to get him to the airport and then Pat Patrick's Learjet to go to Hermann Hospital in Houston, Texas. There was no way I was going to risk leaving a driver at the mercy of the Mexican hospitals in 1980. I had learned years earlier to have an alternate plan ready in case of unexpected weather, failed expectations, sick or injured personnel, or malfunctioning equipment.

I was not happy with this plan, but it was the only choice I had. I took my seat next to Edwards for the start of the race. Since it was CART's first international event, someone in the small kingdom of senior officials had made the brilliant determination that Edwards and I could chase the field on the first lap as they do in Formula One. Bad idea! In Formula One, it works because they use a specially prepared chase car with a race-tuned engine and suspension. We were in our GMC pick-up truck that was totally stock. Top speed was maybe 100 mph.

The race started with Edwards and me in hot pursuit. As we came through the fourth or fifth turn, I can't remember which, I noticed the blue nose of Bobby Unser's Penske rapidly filling our rear view mirror. We had just entered the backstretch and he had caught us already! I yelled at Steve who quickly darted off course to the right. The field thundered by as we watched in stunned disbelief. Needless to say it would be a long time before we tried that again. Unser went on to win the race and thankfully we had no serious incidents.

That night, we attended a big celebration sponsored by the Mexican government. It was held at the President's palace with about 2,000 people in attendance. The waiters were doling out tequila in small shot glasses before dinner. My wife and I were sitting at a table with the Unsers and Al and I had begun to drink the tequila in earnest. We were matching each other shot for shot, first with the tiny glasses then graduating to a cocktail-sized glass. People were watching us expectantly.

After we had consumed several ounces of tequila, the MC unexpectedly called for Al to come to the stage to accept an award. Unser looked at me through glassy eyes and remarked very slowly:

"You go!"

"No way!" I said.

"Karen, you go!"

"No way!" she said.

Al, with some help from the rest of the table, pulled himself from his chair and stumbled to the stage, where he accepted his award for second place. Everyone at the table congratulated him, had some more tequila, and somehow managed to finish dinner.

As we were staggering out of the palace to go back to the hotel, Unser and I stopped to marvel at the government flower beds. Simultaneously, we both had an overwhelming urge to urinate. Not wanting to delay the ride back to the hotel, we began to relieve ourselves on the flowers planted so neatly along the path leading from the palace. We learned later that this was considered a federal offense. Thankfully, we avoided jail and left Mexico City the next morning with the worst headache imaginable. I have not touched tequila since, nor will I ever. Mexico truly *was* different.

Chapter 8

THE RIDE

D uring the winter of 1981, Jon Potter threw a party at his home in Indianapolis during the Christmas holidays. The party was held to celebrate the end of the race season and life in general. Potter had graciously invited Diane and me to attend. While at the party, I became privy to a conversation among some of the drivers, led by Indy champion Bobby Unser. He was expounding on the many virtues of a motorcycle ride he had enjoyed the previous fall. The ride he was referring to was the now famous Colorado 500, the brainchild of Wally Dallenbach and a New Jersey buddy of his named Sherm Cooper. Dallenbach and Cooper had become good friends while racing super-modifieds on the tough tracks in and around Trenton, New Jersey. The two friends had decided to take their motorcycles to Colorado to explore the mountain ranges in and around Aspen in the fall of 1974. They thought the experience so extraordinary they wanted to share it with some of their friends.

Their first invitational ride was held in 1975 and included Dallenbach and Cooper, along with the Unser brothers and five other friends from New Jersey. The nine crazies left Trenton on motorcycles for Colorado in late August. For five days they traversed the rugged mountain trails and fire roads throughout central and southern Colorado. Crazy, adventuresome, or both, they rode on street legal enduro bikes with regular tires, not dirt bikes with knobby tires. Wrestling a made-for-the-highway motorcycle over the 13,000-foot peaks of Colorado was an exhilarating experience, to say the least. Word of their ride soon spread rapidly throughout the Indy racing world and the Colorado 500 was born.

Bobby Unser went on and on about 'The Ride' and I became more and more enthralled. By the end of the evening, I had managed to procure an invitation for the following year. Little did anyone know I had never been on anything bigger than a 50cc Honda scooter. Also, I had never been over mountains taller than the Smokies, and that was in a car with my father at the wheel.

I was determined to go, however, regardless of my horrific lack of experience. These were race drivers and I wanted to be with them. My father had talked me out of being a race driver myself halfway through medical school, probably a good move, but I still had an urge to go fast and to be challenged. The ride offered an opportunity to do just that. I needed to find a bike.

One warm, sunny day in July I went to the local motorcycle store. There, I bought the biggest, meanest dirt bike I could afford. My selection was based primarily on the cool graphics. The only stroke I knew anything about was a bad thing that happened to some people when they grew old. I had no idea what a powerband was or what it was used for. The bike I chose was a two-stroke, 450cc Kawasaki, a bad-assed motocross bike! I was warned repeatedly by the dealer to take it easy. I think he could tell by looking at me that I was something less than a novice.

I financed the bike for as long as the law allowed and somehow managed to ride the thing home from the dealership without crashing. I considered that feat alone pretty phenomenal considering my lack of experience. The bike had awesome power; I was getting really excited!

The second night of ownership, even though I was on call for the hospital, I decided to take my new bike out for practice. It was a beautiful summer evening in mid-July. Diane and I lived on Morse Reservoir, a lake surrounded by a big levee just north of Indianapolis. I knew I would have to climb some very steep hills when I got to the Rockies, so I lined up for an assault on the levee some 40 feet above me.

The levee in Noblesville, Indiana resembled the mountains around Aspen, Colorado about as much as Britney Spears resembles

Rosie O'Donnell. I floored the big green machine. It accelerated instantly and I rocketed to the top of the hill. I was just a-flyin'! I had no idea how fast I was going or how much room I would have once I got to the top. It was a moot point because I blew by the summit, flying into space some 40 feet above the jagged rocks below. I was fucked! There was nowhere to go but down.

I managed to kick the bike away from me while still in mid-air. It landed in the lake with the engine running at full revs. The throttle grip had stuck in the mud on impact and it was wide open. I, unfortunately, landed hard on my tailbone on the rocks a few feet from the motorcycle. I heard my chest crack ominously when I hit the hard stone. My helmet was knocked from my head after making contact with a particularly big rock. I remained conscious, but was in severe pain. Every time I took a breath there was a crunching sound inside my ribcage, not unlike the noise made by a motel ice machine.

A young couple out walking their baby had seen me emerge from behind the levee like Evel Knievel at Caesar's Palace. The man immediately rushed to my side offering his assistance. The bike was still running at full tilt on its side in the lake, spewing water and sand into the evening sky. It was quite a scene.

With the couple's help, I slowly stood up and limped to their car. Their baby, incidentally, was laughing hysterically at me the entire time. I stupidly refused their offer to call for an ambulance so they graciously drove me, crouched painfully in the backseat with the baby, to nearby Riverview Hospital.

Riverview was not unlike the little hospital in Winchester, Indiana. It was small, simple, understaffed, and not in the same league as Methodist Hospital. X-rays revealed several broken ribs and a fractured tailbone. I also had multiple areas of road rash but nothing important seemed to be injured. The fact remained that I couldn't move very fast and it hurt like hell to take a deep breath.

I wasn't there long. I signed out of the hospital against medical advice shortly after midnight when an old battleaxe nurse kept waking me up to ask if I knew who I was. Once awake, she would take my pulse and blood pressure. I told her that if I could speak coherently my blood pressure was just fine and, yes I knew who I was. She and I didn't quite see eye to eye.

I went home early that morning after filling out all of the necessary paperwork. Diane rented a hospital bed and, as I lay in it staring at the ceiling, I couldn't help wonder if 'The Ride' might be a major mistake. It was only four weeks away!

At the end of that time, I was determined as ever to go to Colorado even though I had not been anywhere near my dirt bike since the crash. I flew to Aspen with Wally, following CART's August race in Milwaukee. We met Sherm Cooper in the Aspen airport and drove together to Wally's ranch in Basalt. I was immediately overwhelmed. I had never seen mountains that big before. I couldn't imagine riding anything over them. Sherm asked me where I had been riding lately as he had just returned from a *National Geographic* trip touring South Africa. He said he was going on to Costa Rica after Wally's ride to explore that beautiful country for another magazine. I told him I rode a lot around Noblesville, Indiana.

Sherm was a really cool guy. With his bushy white beard he looked like Santa Claus, but hardened by years of traveling on motorcycles all over the world. When we arrived at Dallenbach's ranch many of the drivers were there; Bobby and Al Unser, Al Unser Jr., Pancho Carter, Rick Mears, Wally Dallenbach Jr., Parnelli Jones, Dan Gurney, Roger Penske, Sir Jack Brabham, Geoff Brabham, famed dirt rider Malcolm Smith, stuntmen Stan Barrett and Walker Evans, and on and on. I didn't tell anyone that the road in from Aspen had scared me a little.

My big green bike had been shipped to the ranch earlier and I was ready to attack the mountains. Problem was I couldn't get my leg over the seat without help. My tailbone was still excruciatingly sore. Also, once I did get on the bike, I couldn't negotiate Wally's gravel driveway. I had never ridden on gravel before and never over any big rocks. I was in deep shit!

Wally's yard the next morning looked like the pit area of the world's biggest motorcycle race. Every conceivable type of dirt bike was represented. The riders had their bikes in various stages of disassembly, fine tuning them for their assault on the mountains. Most of the riders spent the day before the actual ride racing up and down the Frying Pan river valley and into the mountains behind Wally's house. I was afraid to go anyplace. I spent the entire day hanging out with the guys in the yard while my anxiety level rose dramatically. I needed a crash course on dirt bike riding. Pancho Carter and Al Sr., thankfully, took some time to teach me at least a few fundamentals.

The morning of 'The Ride' dawned bright and clear. I was nauseous. After Franklin Graham, the then-young son of the Reverend Billy Graham, gave the invocation, the mayor of Basalt, Colorado gave the command to start engines. Dallenbach looked at me and just shook his head. Karen Unser remarked to my wife:

"He looks so frail!"

I lived up to my appearance. Within an hour I was lost in a creek deep in the forest. I had no clue that the Rockies had been called the Rockies because they were basically composed of big, loose rocks. To me it was like trying to ride over a pile of bowling balls. All I could think about as I sat there by the creek was the grizzly bear in the Coors beer commercial who comes down to the river to get a drink. I was petrified!

After what seemed like a lifetime Gay Smith, one of the expert riders, showed up. I had positioned myself between the edge of the creek and my motorcycle just in case the bear was near by. Smith, a good friend of Dallenbach's was, I suspect, assigned the task of specifically watching over me. He was another racer, having driven in the famous Pike's Peak hillclimb for a number of years. He helped me get my bike restarted and I followed him to the top of Taylor Pass. This was a significant accomplishment considering the fact that none of my four extremities was ever in contact with the bike at the same time. Once on top of the mountain, the view from 13,000 feet was spectacular! I was too nervous to enjoy it.

After a brief stop on Taylor Pass, all the riders were supposed to meet for lunch at a cabin very high in the mountains. I was the last rider to arrive at the cabin. Dallenbach looked at me again and said with no facial expression at all:

"I can't believe you're here!"

That raised my confidence level to a new high. I then made another huge mistake. I got off the bike. After lunch, I wasn't able to get back on and required the help of one of the other riders. I shudder to think what he must have thought. I promptly fell behind again as soon as we left the cabin and was hopelessly lost within minutes. I had no clue where I was. It soon began to grow dark and windy as a summer storm approached.

This time, after being lost for nearly three hours, I was saved by an elderly couple who were out four-wheel-driving for the afternoon. They looked at me in a suspicious sort of way, but, after hearing my tail of woe, allowed me to get into their Jeep. I left the motorcycle behind, not caring if I ever saw it again.

The old couple drove me effortlessly into the little town of Silverton where I met up with the rest of the guys to spend the night. I soon discovered that abandoning your motorcycle was tantamount to deserting your horse. The other riders couldn't believe it! I had no idea where I was when I left it, so I was no help in finding it. The evil machine was discovered the next day by a group of riders who happened upon it just outside of town. They loaded it into one of the chase trucks and I became reacquainted with it that evening.

For the remainder of the trip I rode in a truck driven by Bob Larson, a friend of Dallenbach's and a local resident of Basalt. Larson and I spent the day rescuing other broken down and lost riders. I managed an occasional short ride on my bike as we traversed the mountains. I slowly gained more confidence. Unser Sr., out of pity, succeeded in teaching me how to ride respectably and I was able to return for nine more years. 'The Ride' produced many lasting friendships that remain to this day. In the early years of 'The Ride' it served as a common thread among many of the racing drivers. It was an event designed to have fun, be challenging, relaxing, and to heal any emotional wounds that had accumulated during the season.

I wasn't totally useless that first year. Jack Murray, a captain for Continental Airlines and crewman for Johnny Rutherford, sustained a deep gash in his knee when a rock, ejected from beneath another bike, bull's-eyed his kneecap. I met Murray as he hobbled into the lobby bar in Silverton. I was there, hanging out with a group of the other riders drinking whiskey, and watching Roger Penske play liar's poker with hundred dollar bills. Murray was bleeding profusely from his lacerated knee. We had no suture material available, so I asked the barmaid if she happened to have any thread. She said she had some beautiful light blue thread in her purse. Anesthetic was provided compliments of Jack Daniels.

After he and I had consumed most of the bottle, I sutured the really nasty cut using the barmaid's pretty blue thread and one of her needles. Jack was real proud of his new scar and later enjoyed showing it to barmaids all over the southern Rockies. The cut miraculously healed without getting infected and the scar was minimal. On subsequent rides, we would carry much more first aid equipment.

The number of injuries sustained by the riders that year was substantial. One concussion occurred as a result of a rider trying to drive his bike through a cow. Steve Edwards was also on his first ride, and he and I were kept fairly busy tending to the wounded. Everyone survived, even oilman Bobby Hillin.

Hillin, you'll remember, was Unser Sr.'s car owner and a big oil tycoon from Texas. He had never been in the wilderness and he had no clue what to do if he got lost. He managed to get hopelessly lost at the end of the third day. We had finished with dinner that night and it became apparent that Hillin wasn't going to make it to the hotel. A search party was quickly formed, led by world champion rider, Malcolm Smith. Malcolm was acknowledged as the best all-around dirt rider in the world. He had won the International Six Day Trials on several occasions and had just returned from an endurance race in South Africa. He left the motel in the dark, holding a pen light between his teeth. Edwards and I were put on alert status. We waited for what seemed like a very long time.

Hillin had become separated from Al Sr. at some point during the day after taking a wrong turn into a blind canyon. It had soon grown dark. Following repeated attempts to find his way out, he simply sat down by his bike, exhausted, and waited. He had sufficient fuel in his tank and several matches, but it never occurred to him to start a fire. He just laid there and waited, as the night grew colder and colder.

Around 11 o'clock Smith, still holding the penlight in his teeth, found the shivering Hillin huddled next to his motorcycle. He was barely coherent. His skin in the dim light was a pale shade of blue. The air temperature had fallen to below 30 degrees. He was markedly hypothermic.

The rescue party brought the nearly frozen rider back to the hotel, where I gradually warmed him up with liquids and blankets. Thankfully, he was able to join us at breakfast the next morning. He was dressed and ready to ride. Big Al scolded him for the duration of the trip. 'The Ride' truly was a wonderful experience and generated tremendous camaraderie among the participants.

Tragedy, however, would soon strike. Art Lamey, the very likable Champion spark plug representative in Indycars, and a good friend to everyone in racing, would succumb to a fatal heart attack on the top of Taylor Pass. Crippen, Edwards, Stan Barrett, three other Hollywood stuntmen, and I attempted to resuscitate him at an altitude of 13,000 feet. CPR was excruciatingly difficult at that altitude. We performed it in tandem, with each man lasting only a few pumps on the chest. We had been at it for more than 40 minutes when we tragically ran out of oxygen and IV fluids. The rescue helicopter, trying to find us, had become lost in the fog and arrived too late. Art died doing what he loved to do and a memorial currently rests on top of Taylor Pass, placed there in his honor by the men of 'The Ride'.

Franklin Graham, Dennis Agajanian and I rode sadly back

to the ranch to tell his wife what had happened. I think she somehow already knew. The Ride lost a great comrade and the sport a great gentleman. Many more Colorado 500s would occur, with any number of tall tales and true. I credit Dallenbach and his Ride for instilling in me a love of motorcycles and the people who ride them. The 30th anniversary was held in 2005. Not as many Indycar drivers go now because the racing schedule is too tight, and the sport is such big business. During those first 10 or 12 years, however, Dallenbach's Ride was a common thread throughout the sport of Indycar racing and a topic of conversation for the entire year. It became obvious to me that race drivers, motocross riders, and other motorsports participants have much in common. They all started very young and had gained the ability to become one with whatever machine they were riding or driving. Unless you're like them you have no chance to compete on their level.

Chapter 9

THE MAGICIAN

During the 1981 500 Mile Race, Dr. Bock and I were still working together on the race track at Indianapolis. Bock was stationed in the Safety Truck at the north end of the track between Turns 3 and 4, and I was in the truck at the south end between Turns 1 and 2. Dr. Hanna was at his usual post in the infield care center. Bock had taken over as Medical Director of USAC when I jumped ship and moved to CART in 1979. USAC had continued to sanction the Indy 500, with CART sanctioning all of the other races. The Speedway's management still allowed me to work on the race track since the vast majority of the drivers in the race were from the CART series. Many of the USAC stalwarts, however, considered me to be a traitor and the situation was becoming strained. Bock and I worked well together in spite of all the bickering and behind-the-back talking, sharing the responsibility for on-track medical care.

Late in the race the 'Flying Hawaiian', Danny Ongais, was very much in contention. Ongais was a nearly pure-blooded Hawaiian, having come upon the Indycar scene from Southern California after doing well in both drag and motorcycle racing. He was a man of few words, doing most of his talking with his racecar. He was extremely fast, but not always under good control.

Just past the halfway point in the race, while exiting Turn 3, he suddenly lost control and pounded the outside retaining wall. He came to rest with the right side of his car smeared against the concrete midway into the short stretch. Bock arrived at the crash scene within seconds; my truck arrived shortly thereafter. Ongais was unconscious with both of his legs protruding grotesquely from the car's mangled front end. Bock and I quickly stabilized his neck and secured his airway. We carefully extricated him with the help of the firemen, and airlifted him to Methodist Hospital, not taking time to do anything else. Taking time to start an intravenous line at the scene is usually unnecessary. It only delays the extrication as well as the event. There is ample time to place an IV in the ambulance, or in the care center, since it usually takes no more than five minutes to get there. On the highway, an injured person may have sat hemorrhaging for several minutes to an hour or more before help would arrive at the scene.

On duty in the Methodist Hospital emergency room that day was a brash young orthopedic surgeon who had recently completed a spine surgery fellowship in Toronto, Canada. He enjoyed taking care of trauma patients when not operating on someone's backbone and was a huge race fan. Like Bock and me, he was an Indiana native. His name was Dr. Terry Trammell.

Trammell was stuck in the emergency room on the day Ongais crashed. He was there because he was the youngest physician in his group, therefore the low man on the totem pole. Most of his partners were, in fact, at the race. He met Ongais when they unloaded him from the ambulance.

The right leg was damaged more than the left. There was a large, gaping wound with an obvious open fracture. Ongais required immediate surgery to save the limb. The fracture was a dirty one, with bone protruding from the wound. Ongais was immediately rushed to the operating room where Dr. Trammell did a masterful job of reconstructing the right leg. During the surgery, Trammell was surprised to find that Ongais was actually missing a large chunk of bone from his tibia. Searching the wound, the lost piece of bone was nowhere to be found. Amazingly, the track's clean-up crew discovered the errant piece of bone the next day. It had been forcefully ejected through the driver's triple-layered firesuit on impact and had then sailed over the retaining wall, lodging itself in the dirt embankment on the other side. A large hole in Ongais' driver's suit bore testament to the huge forces that are involved in a 200 mph crash into concrete.

Trammell managed to save the leg from amputation using recently developed blood vessel sparing techniques. These had previously been the purview of vascular surgeons only. Ongais recovered from his injuries with the right leg about an inch shorter than the left. He returned to race for many more years. Dr. Trammell, as word spread quickly throughout the racing community, would soon become practically every American racing driver's orthopedic surgeon of choice. Robin Miller, the very knowledgeable race reporter for the *Indianapolis Star* at the time, called Trammell the 'Magician'. The name stuck. Trammell has since operated on more racing drivers in the world than any other 20 physicians combined. He has continually developed seat-of-the-pants techniques to save a limb or to replace shattered boney pieces in such a way that a driver can race again. He and I soon became close friends, sharing a love for the sport of auto racing. He is an esteemed colleague and friend to this day.

Chapter 10

A.J. Crashes Again

The late 70s through 1981 were relatively safe years for CART. Many spectacular accidents occurred, but remarkably there were no fatalities. Basically, we had been lucky. One very serious incident involving the legendary A.J. Foyt did stand out, however. It occurred during the Michigan 500 in 1981. Michigan International Speedway is a two-mile, high-banked race track. It is situated in the Irish Hills district of southern Michigan, a low-income resort area roughly an hour's drive from Detroit airport.

Like the track in Phoenix, Michigan International Speedway used steel barriers rather than the more expensive concrete wall for impact containment. Not only the inside, but the outside of the track was surrounded by the dangerous stuff! Merle Bettenhausen, middle son of the late Tony Bettenhausen, crashed there in 1972 and had most of his right arm amputated by the wicked steel rails. In spite of this injury, and a number of other injuries at race tracks around the world, steel barriers were still in common usage.

A.J. was leading the race when he crashed heavily while exiting the second turn. He smashed broadside into the outer barrier. The car slid to a stop right up against the retaining wall, a short distance from the initial point of impact. When we arrived at the scene, Edwards and I found A.J. slumped unconscious over the steering wheel. Three separate streams of blood were flowing from beneath his car. They flowed down the steep banking and into the infield grass.

Usually a big wreck like this attracts all of the track workers to the scene like maggots, whether they're needed or not. Edwards and I were surprised to find that we were the only ones at the car. The rest of the workers were milling about, picking up debris and seeming to shy away from the wreck. The reason was simple. This was A.J. Foyt! A living hero to most of the safety guys. The sight of him slumped over unconscious and bleeding was too much for them to handle.

Arriving on the scene of a crash immediately after the crash occurs is unique for on-track rescue workers. The only similar situation that comes to mind is a runway crash at an airport with an immediate response by the field's firecrew. Our Safety Trucks normally arrive on the scene just as the wrecked car or cars are rolling to a stop. On the highway, medics usually don't arrive until several minutes or perhaps hours after the crash. They rarely, if ever, see an actual crash occur right there in front of them. Likewise, they rarely know or recognize the victims. We arrive in seconds, and we know most of the drivers well. In fact, Dr. Trammell and I have socialized with many of them on a regular basis. This single fact is probably the most frightening aspect of working the races. No one wants to see a good friend injured or hurt in any way.

Foyt's right arm was nearly amputated by the sharp edges of the steel barrier. He was bleeding heavily from his brachial artery, the big one in the upper arm. It was a spiral type of laceration, the result of his arm being twisted and squeezed as the car's body ground it against the sharp edge of the barrier. Had the laceration remained in one plane his arm would have been completely severed. Edwards and I commented later that it was actually easier to work this crash than some others because we were not hampered by 'too many' hands. The extrication was still difficult, mostly because of A.J.'s size. We managed to get him out without doing any more harm and placed him into the waiting ambulance. IVs were started to replace his lost fluids.

In addition to the arm injury, Foyt had also sustained a moderately severe concussion. He had remained unconscious throughout the entire extrication process. I jumped in the ambulance with him and told the driver to go straight to the heliport. The flight crew and I had some difficulty squeezing him into Penske's corporate helicopter. Foyt had grown heavier over the years and had literally to be wedged between the plush upholstery of the chopper's leather covered seats and the ceiling. Once in, I stuffed the IV bag between his belly and the padded ceiling and sent him on his way to the University of Michigan Hospital in Ann Arbor. He was still unconscious.

He was seen in the emergency room on arrival, and later admitted to the intensive care unit. Foyt had awakened somewhat during the flight and had begun to argue with the flight crew about getting out of town. By the time he arrived in the emergency room, he was fully awake.

I drove straight to the hospital as soon as the race was over and tried in vain to speak with the doctors taking care of him. They didn't want to hear what I had to say. I was still in my CART official's uniform and didn't look like a doctor to them. University doctors, by nature, are a highly suspicious group and many don't think too highly of race track doctors trying to give them any meaningful information. As a consequence, they didn't allow me access to Foyt once he was admitted. These rather arrogant doctors thus remained unaware of some meaningful details of the crash. They were not aware that Foyt had been unconscious for more than 15 minutes. They admitted him for observation without obtaining a CT scan of his brain.

The university doctors released him on his insistence the next morning, allowing him to fly home in a friend's private jet. This was not a good thing to do. I later heard from a friend of his, now deceased, that when he arrived in Houston, he began complaining of severe headaches and had developed double vision. Rightfully worried, his family contacted a physician friend who quickly referred him to a neurosurgeon.

Reportedly, the CT scan that should have been performed in Michigan was finally ordered. A.J.'s friend told me it revealed a small blood clot on A.J.'s brain. This type of clot is called a subdural hematoma. It is caused when blood collects between the brain and its thick covering membrane called the dura. It is almost always the result of head trauma. Had the jet depressurized on its way to Houston, the clot could easily have expanded, jamming the brain through the base of the skull and possibly killing Foyt instantly. University hospitals, I sadly discovered, are not always the best place to be for acute trauma. They don't often see acute trauma in the large numbers that are seen in big city trauma centers.

After Foyt's crash, I never allowed a driver with a documented loss of consciousness to escape without a CT scan of his brain. Also, as a result of that accident, I was finally able to convince CART to require promoters, even Roger Penske, to hire true medical evacuation helicopters for the transportation of seriously injured drivers. Even though they are expensive, there is no substitute for a properly equipped and manned aircraft.

Chapter 11

DEATH PAYS US A VISIT

The excellent safety record enjoyed by CART during its first three seasons was to change suddenly in 1982. During an attempt to qualify for the Indy 500, Gordon Smiley, a cocky young driver from Texas, was determined to break 200 mph or die trying. Several veteran drivers, including Al Unser Sr. and Johnny Rutherford, had warned him that he was in way over his head, driving all wrong for the Speedway. Smiley was a road racer and was used to counter-steering his car to avoid a crash if the rear wheels broke traction.

On his final warm-up lap prior to qualifying, Smiley pushed way too hard as he drove deep into Turn 3. He lost the rear end of the car and tried to correct it by turning right, into the slide. This is taboo on an oval. The car never completely lost traction due to the sliding skirts, allowed in 1982 for added ground effects. He plowed straight into the wall as a result. If he had locked the brakes his car would have likely spun harmlessly into the infield grass or simply come to an eventual stop.

He hit the concrete so hard it appeared to some observers that he had actually tried to drive his car through the wall. Both front wheels left identical black footprints on the stark white concrete; a testament to the nearly 90-degree impact. It was unlike any previous Indycar crash. On the television replay, Nikki, my 12-year-old daughter, said it looked as if the wall had swallowed the car up and then spat it back out. It was the most devastating crash ever witnessed at the Speedway.

Smiley's car flew into the air after impact, soaring some 15 feet above the pavement. It clobbered the angled debris fence. What remained of the car then flipped end-over-end repeatedly, until it finally came to rest more than a quarter of a mile downstream. Only the twisted seat, with Smiley still strapped inside, remained intact. The rest of the car was scattered in small pieces throughout the north end of the Speedway.

I was in the Safety Truck as usual that year and arrived at the scene with USAC Safety Director, Jack Gilmore. While rushing to the car, I noticed small splotches of a peculiar gray substance marking a trail on the asphalt leading up to the driver. When I reached the car, I was shocked to see that Smiley's helmet was gone, along with the top of his skull. He had essentially been scalped by the debris fence. The material on the race track was most of his brain. His helmet, due to massive centrifugal force, was literally pulled from his head on impact. It was tossed some distance from the car. When we found it the chinstrap was still fastened.

All Gilmore and I could do was cover the body with a fire blanket and respectfully transfer him to the waiting ambulance. I rode to the care center with the body. On the way in I performed a cursory examination and realized that nearly every bone in his body was shattered. He had a gaping wound in his side that looked as if he had been attacked by a large shark. I had never seen such trauma.

Jack and I had hoped to shield Smiley's body from the eager ring of predatory photographers who always seem to multiply on the first day of qualifications for Indy. In spite of our efforts, one of them managed to get some grizzly pictures that later appeared in print much to everyone's disgust.

That May was Dr. Bock's first year as Medical Director of the Speedway. Dr. Hanna had died suddenly the previous winter following a ruptured abdominal aortic aneurysm. Bock was the logical choice to take over the Speedway Medical Team as he had remained in USAC when I took the position in CART. He did not deserve such an initiation. Barbara Smiley, Gordon's wife, was at the track that day and was in the care center when I arrived with the body. Bock and I gave her the tragic news together. Death had not visited the Speedway since 1973.

Smiley's death, since we declared him at the track, was made a coroner's case to comply with state law. This caused a major disruption in the care center, turning the whole event into an even worse nightmare. Operations within the little hospital came to a virtual standstill while waiting for the coroner to arrive. Ironically, he was caught in a major traffic jam, the result of people still trying to get into the Speedway to see qualifications.

Bock and I made a major decision as soon as the coroner and the body left the building. From that day on, nobody would die at the race track unless they were decapitated or incinerated in their car. This unwritten rule soon became dogma throughout the entire racing world. Unfortunately, it has been invoked too many times.

Smiley's death threw all of us into a state of shock. I had actually entertained the idea that the sport had become relatively safe and this kind of crash would never be seen again. Earlier, one of the drivers had even complained to me that I had been touting the safety angle way too much. He knew better. We had been rudely awakened. Racing was still very dangerous! The veteran drivers shrugged it off as a novice mistake.

"If he had only listened," they said.

The show, without Gordon Smiley, went on as it always does. The race was completed two weeks later without any serious mishaps, and the circus left for the next race. Three weeks after Smiley's death we were in Milwaukee for the famous Milwaukee Mile, a race that traditionally follows Indy. During Saturday's afternoon practice session, Edwards and I were sitting, relaxed, at our post just past pit out. There were three minutes to go in the session and Steve and I were already discussing where we would like to eat dinner that evening. Practice was scheduled to go until six o'clock.

Jim Hickman, a wealthy car dealer from Atlanta with very limited experience in Indycar racing, suddenly shot past our station without slowing down at all for the first turn. The roar from his engine told us that his throttle was wide open! The result sent him straight into the wall. The car exploded into several small pieces.

Edwards and I were on the scene in less than 15 seconds. Hickman was bleeding profusely from his nose and mouth. He was completely unresponsive and barely breathing. We protected his airway by placing a tube in his nose and starting oxygen. He had obviously sustained a very bad head injury. The pupils of his eyes were widely dilated. They did not react to light. We loaded him quickly into the ambulance. I jumped in beside him for the short ride to the trauma center. I had seen enough severe head injuries to know that his chances of survival were very slim. Surprisingly, he was still breathing on his own so I continued full life support.

Hickman arrived in the emergency room with stable vital signs and obvious severe brain damage. He continued to breathe on his own until four o'clock the following morning. He was diagnosed officially brain dead by the local neurosurgeon shortly thereafter. We had suddenly lost two drivers in three weeks. Our luck had run out. Death in racing, as in nearly all sports, can raise its ugly head at any moment.

During the investigation of the crash it was discovered that Hickman's team had mounted his 'kill switch' on the dashboard of the car instead of on the steering wheel where it should have been; too far away to reach in a panic situation. Hickman had kept both of his hands glued to the steering wheel trying to negotiate the corner. Following the crash investigation, the location for these switches with a mount on the steering wheel was made mandatory. There, they could be reached quickly with a thumb or finger. NASCAR, the largest racing organization in the country, surprisingly didn't address this concern until the death of Richard Petty's grandson Adam in a similar type of crash at the New Hampshire Speedway in 2001.

Until 1982, safety innovations were usually made in response to a fatal crash. This was true for all of the major sanctioning bodies.

Following such crashes, the changes made to the cars, or to the rules, were usually knee-jerk reactions that seemed to make sense at the time, but were not necessarily the result of good scientific studies. A proactive approach to safety was virtually non-existent. No one scientifically studied the plight of the racing driver with regard to safety. Most scientists felt the sport, if it truly was a sport, had nothing to offer the outside world. A world unto itself, automobile racing was left to fend for itself outside of academia.

After the deaths of Smiley and Hickman, Dr. Trammell brought up the idea of documenting and eventually publishing our accident and injury statistics in a real medical journal. We had been collecting data internally for some time in order to spot our own injury trends and to identify the causes of injury. By publishing the data, we would make this information available to other physicians and health care providers interested in racing safety. We saw no reason to keep the information to ourselves. No one in racing had ever published data on crash and injury statistics before. Terry and I felt strongly that we could help improve the safety of racecars everywhere with the data we were collecting.

Our first paper was published in 1984. The study appeared in *Physician and Sports Medicine*, not a peer-reviewed journal, but rather a so-called 'throwaway', the type of journal doctors read in the bathroom. But it was a start. In our original study, we showed that orthopedic injuries accounted for 89% of all the injuries sustained during the period studied. Head injuries, though often severe, comprised only 10%. Surprisingly, internal injuries such as a ruptured spleen or a lacerated liver were less than 1% of the total. The injury distribution we uncovered in CART is very different from that reported on our highways. Passenger car crashes frequently result in severe internal chest and abdominal injuries. So much so, that the primary focus in major trauma centers after the head and neck is on the chest and abdomen.

The scarcity of internal injuries in motorsports remains just as true today as it was then. The driver's torso is so well restrained by the six-point belt system that the internal organs are very well protected. The driver is anchored firmly by his seatbelt, shoulder harness, and crotch straps. By anchoring the pelvis, restraining the chest, and preventing any submarine motion of the body on impact, the internal organs are pretty secure. The lack of adequate restraint in passenger cars on the other hand, allows the body to move around violently inside the vehicle during a crash. As a result, there are often many secondary impacts with parts of the vehicle, each capable of producing a large variety of injuries.

Our study uncovered two primary areas of concern for us. One, we needed to learn how to prevent, or at least mitigate severe distal (foot and ankle) orthopedic injuries; and two, we needed a better way to protect the head. The feet and legs during a crash were allowed to bounce around freely inside the car, coming into contact with a variety of internal chassis parts. The brake, clutch and throttle pedals produced a number of foot and ankle fractures. The head and neck were also subjected to a variety of extreme accelerations after impact as the car responded violently to the forces of the crash. Focal injuries, such as skull fracture or contusion, were rare. Most head injuries were the result of rotational forces that usually caused concussion or, if extreme, would cause what is referred to as a diffuse axonal injury. DAI is a form of severe shearing injury to the brain that is often fatal.

Amazingly, 48% of the drivers in our initial study had never been injured at all! Mario Andretti, probably the greatest American racing driver of all time, was one of these. Mario had raced cars since he was 13 years old. He had raced in every kind of vehicle imaginable. He had won the Formula One title in Europe as well as both the Indy 500 and the Daytona 500 in the United States. He raced sprint cars, midget cars, Indycars, stock cars and F1 cars, yet by 1984 he had never suffered so much as a broken finger. He holds records in every series he contested, but the fact he never suffered a serious injury is truly one of his most remarkable accomplishments.

The vast majority of orthopedic injuries in our study were to the feet and ankles. This was largely due to the exposure of the lower extremities in frontal impacts. Dr. Trammell was kept busy operating throughout the 80s with a steady influx of drivers bearing shattered feet and ankles. The number of drivers who had sustained crippling injuries was growing exponentially during this period and the sport was getting a bad reputation as a result. Something had to be done quickly to curtail this epidemic of broken bones.

CART's technical committee, along with the engineers, met on numerous occasions during the mid-80s. Using their engineering skills and much of our data, they made a number of changes to the cars. The nosecone was strengthened, the driver was moved further back in the car, and an additional bulkhead was added in front of the driver's feet. The result of these changes was a defined footbox and a definite decrease in the severity of foot and ankle injuries. This decrease was made readily apparent in our second study, published in 1989. It showed that lower extremity injuries had decreased to 60% of the total. There were still plenty of injuries to keep Dr. Trammell busy, but most of them were not as disabling as in the past.

As a result of the decrease in orthopedic injuries, head injuries had increased to nearly 40% of the total. We were not having more head injuries, we were simply having fewer orthopedic injuries. Fortunately, most of the head injuries were relatively minor in nature. Typically, a driver would be knocked unconscious or dazed on impact, with a full recovery one to three minutes after the crash. A driver was said to have 'had his bell rung' if he sustained this type of head injury. At the time, we considered such a driver lucky the injury wasn't a lot worse. Back then, we didn't know the consequences of too many minor head injuries.

Trammell and I learned a good lesson regarding mild head injury when Johnny Rutherford had a spectacular crash during the 1983 Phoenix race. Initially, he seemed to be fine as he easily climbed out of his wrecked car. He was able to converse with the rescue team and he made sense. Trammell was the doctor at the scene of this particular crash and he allowed Rutherford to walk across the track on his own. Once in the infield, JR got lost trying to find his motorhome. Gary Gerould, one of the TV announcers looking for an interview, came upon the bewildered driver as he wandered aimlessly through the maze of parked vehicles. By this time, he didn't know which end was up. The interview was largely unintelligible. Embarrassed by this fiasco, we made a rule that anyone who crashed on an oval was to be taken straight to the medical center for a period of observation. If there was any deterioration in their condition they were sent on to the trauma center for a complete neurological evaluation and CT scan.

The fact that injuries experienced in racing are so different from those seen on our highways is the primary reason that a dedicated medical team is a must for any motorsports series. Also, where possible, it is advisable to have a dedicated safety team of firemen and paramedics. Using the same individuals to do driver extrications leads to greater coordination and speed, as well as a decrease in the likelihood of causing further injury during the extrication. After a bad crash, the driver is often found tangled in a wide variety of exotic racecar parts and is physically unable to get out of the cockpit. Not knowing what those parts are made of, or what they are connected to, can easily lead to further injury when using the extrication tools. These tools are heavy and difficult to control. Aimlessly cutting stuff to get the driver out of the car can easily lead to an inadvertent amputation.

Having the same medical team attending the injured drivers also decreases the likelihood that injuries unique to motorsports will be missed. There are a number of soft tissue injuries and occult fractures that occur to race drivers that are rarely if ever seen in highway travelers. These injuries will be described as we go along in this book. All racing crashes by definition meet so-called 'trauma criteria'. As such, every driver involved in a crash would be immobilized on a backboard and rushed to the local trauma center if seen by only the local medics. There, the driver could be subjected to a number of expensive, exhaustive, and unnecessary tests looking for injuries that never happen.

Other injuries unique to motorsports would stand a good chance of being missed.

This happened in the late 90s when Mark Blundell, a former British Formula One driver and Indycar winner, crashed during a private test session at the St. Louis race track. He had a severe rear impact that resulted in an immediate collection of blood and tissue fluid in his lower back. Fascinated by this, the doctors in the emergency room missed a significant cervical fracture and allowed Mark to fly home in a private airplane piloted by his friend, P.J. Jones. Luckily, the injury was discovered and treated by his personal physician and no paralysis resulted.

Trammell and I know from experience which drivers are likely to be hurt and which aren't, following a crash. We can determine the likely injuries by knowing what part of the car is damaged and by how much. Our rapid assessment of a crash, which we now do automatically, includes the angle of impact, the speed of the car, and the condition of any obstacle with which the car made contact. We have therefore saved a lot of drivers from a lengthy and unnecessary visit to the emergency room.

Formula One also has a dedicated medical team. Professor Sid Watkins developed a sophisticated system within Formula One beginning in 1978, roughly paralleling the work I was doing in America. He was faced with the challenge of racing in many different countries with a variety of customs and multiple languages. Logistics made a traveling squad of medics and firemen nearly impossible due to the high cost and varying nationalities. As a consequence, Professor Watkins developed a network of extremely competent individuals to internally organize and operate dedicated medical teams at the various Formula One tracks. His partner in this development was Dr. Jean-Jacques Isserman, who would arrive at a venue early to inspect the trauma center of choice and all vehicles, equipment, and personnel involved in potential rescues.

Competing on almost exclusively permanent race tracks hosting multiple annual events, these individuals, trained under Watkins, would return year after year developing the same type of close working relationships with each other as we enjoyed in the CART series. Protocols were developed and standards were put in place by Professor Watkins around the world, the better to care for the Grand Prix drivers. Upon Dr Watkins' retirement in 2004, that work is being continued by my fellow countryman Dr Gary Hartstein.

Another advantage to having a dedicated Safety Team lies in the inherent dangers that lurk in the hostile and energy charged environment of a 'hot' race track. During a yellow condition on the track, traffic does not come to a stop while the rescue workers attend the crash. This is very different from what happens during a highway crash where the police are usually in control of traffic flow by the time the ambulance arrives. Rescue workers on the highway are normally able to perform their rescue duties without the fear of being run over.

During a yellow-flag condition in racing, the cars often don't slow down at all. In fact, timing and scoring officials have pointed out to us that some of the driver's fastest laps have occurred during yellow-flag periods! This can be quite disconcerting and downright hazardous for those attempting an on-track rescue. Dr. Crippen, on one frightening occasion, was forced to jump into the cockpit of the wrecked car of Al Unser Sr. in order to avoid being run over. The car that nearly hit Crippen had lost control after sliding on oil dumped from Unser's car when his engine blew up. Crippen was lucky. Race track savvy, as I call it, is vital in order to survive under these conditions.

Medical and fire personnel having little on-track racing experience are in great danger in such unpredictable surroundings. I have learned over the years to pay particular attention to unusual or strange sounds while trying to concentrate on the extrication of an injured driver. A car whose engine suddenly becomes silent, or a car producing excessive tire noise near the scene can signal a loss of control and impending danger to track rescue personnel.

Without a dedicated team of paramedics, firemen, and doctors, much useful information can also be lost due to an inherent mistrust of local medical personnel that resides within most race drivers. The trust that develops over the years in a dedicated team of physicians helps in gathering all of the information about a crash, as well as the total extent of injuries a driver may have sustained. I learned from Rick Mears, for example, that several drivers had been losing consciousness following relatively minor crashes during testing throughout much of the 80s. This increase in minor head injury occurred at the same time that carbon fiber had replaced aluminum as the principal structural material used in the driver's safety cell. This change in materials resulted in a much stiffer cockpit that included the cockpit rim. Without the 'give' inherent in aluminum, many drivers suffered a minor concussion when their heads made contact with the newly developed, very stiff carbon fiber during an otherwise minor impact.

Mears relayed this information to me following a crash he had while testing a car in Milwaukee. He had crashed in the afternoon, but was totally unaware of it until learning of it during a dinner conversation with his crew. He told me about the incident later that same week and the two of us determined the cause. If Rick hadn't trusted me, who knows how long it would have been before anyone knew what was happening to the drivers? We were able to remedy the situation quickly by padding the cockpit rim with energy-absorbing foam to lessen these secondary impacts. The problem disappeared overnight.

Over the years, the CART drivers drew very close to Dr. Trammell and me. They knew they had two friends to whom they could entrust sensitive information. They knew we would use that information to further safety in a sport that not too long before had been extremely dangerous, if not foolhardy. This familiarity also provided a sense of security for the drivers that would otherwise have been lacking. This same trust and respect was given to Professor Watkins on the other side of the Atlantic.

By the time Terry and I had published our second paper in 1989, we had learned the basic essentials of race driver protection. These essential rules remain as true today as they did then. The key to injury prevention in an open-wheeled racing car is to restrain the driver fully in a very strong, safety cell or 'tub'. The tub then needs to be surrounded by breakaway, energy absorbing parts. The wheels with their rubber tires, the multiple suspension components, and importantly the sidepods of the car, all serve to dissipate kinetic energy during a crash. The sidepods not only absorb energy, but help divert errant pieces of debris away from, and over, a driver's head.

The driver's seat needs to be seamless and supportive with particular attention to support of the shoulders. The 45-degree angle of most open-cockpit car seats is the lowest a seat should recline. All sharp surfaces within the cockpit need to be padded, eliminated, or smoothed off. The pedals need to be as wide as possible and suspension geometry must be such that intrusion into the cockpit is nearly impossible. If these rules are followed then usually, but not always, a spectacularly exploding crash spares injury to the driver.

The crashes that concern us the most are the ones where few parts leave the car on impact. In these crashes, the car suddenly decelerates over a very short time and distance, overwhelming the crushability of the various components. This rapid deceleration, or sudden stop, is the cause of most life-threatening injuries that result from a racing accident. With the energy absorbing structures overwhelmed, too much of the impact's kinetic energy is transmitted to the driver. Their head and neck are the most vulnerable in the modern racing car as they are not as protected, or as well restrained, as the rest of the body. These areas became the focus of intense study and are reserved for discussion later in this book.

Chapter 12

RICK MEARS PROVES HE'S HUMAN AFTER ALL

C ART, thankfully, had no further fatalities in 1982 and had a reasonably good year in 1983. In the summer of 1984 we found ourselves at beautiful, but remote, Sanair Speedway almost 60 miles from Montreal, one of Canada's most handsome and charming cities. During the Friday morning practice session, Rick Mears uncharacteristically lost control of his car coming out of the fourth turn. He had made a sudden cut in front of a couple of cars, clipped one of them, and that sent him rocketing into the steel barrier. No one could remember Rick ever losing control like that. He had crashed before, but it was always due to the loss of control of another driver or something breaking on his car. He crashed heavily. His car came to a stop just 20 feet behind Edwards and me sitting quietly in our Safety Truck.

We were parked, as usual, at pit out facing into the first turn. Race Control dispatched us immediately to the scene. I yelled to Steve to stay put. I had noticed the commotion unfolding behind us in the truck's rearview mirror. I jumped from the truck and ran back to Rick's car. He was slumped over the steering wheel unconscious, with his feet mangled and entrapped in the car's severely damaged front end. The steel barrier had literally ripped the front of the car apart, destroying his feet in the process. The extrication required careful handling in order to cause no further harm. It was a long one. Rick's feet were pinched and tangled in the web of cables and control assemblies housed in the nose of the car.

Edwards and his crew did a masterful job removing him from

the crumpled machine. We carefully placed him in the ambulance, I jumped in, and we started for the hospital in St-Pie, the closest town. We got only as far as the main gate when we suddenly stopped. Two different ambulance attendants strolled slowly up to the window and informed me that the ambulance we were in was only the track ambulance and as such, it could not go out on to the highway. I was dumbfounded!

"Don't worry," they said. "Another ambulance has been summoned and you will just have to wait."

Mears was beginning to stir and starting to moan in pain. He continued to lapse in and out of consciousness as his feet began to swell. The new ambulance finally arrived after several minutes and we headed out on to the highway, but only after the exchange of a few pleasantries between attendants. The long delay had allowed Roger Penske, Mears' car owner, to jump into the ambulance next to me. Great, I really needed that. Penske was determined to accompany his driver to the hospital. Compounding the problem was the fact that the ambulance attendants refused to speak any further English. They sat stoically in the front seat, conversing happily with each other in French.

Mears' feet continued to balloon in size and, by this time, had turned the color of grape jelly. After traveling for about seven miles we again came to a sudden stop. This time we appeared to be in the middle of absolutely nowhere. We were the only vehicle at a remote crossroads somewhere in the Quebec countryside. The scene looked like a drug deal about to come off. Penske looked at me and I looked at him. The two attendants shrugged their shoulders, smiled, and refused to speak to us. Mears was still unconscious, occasionally mumbling incoherently while his feet continued to swell. Penske and I were getting really agitated trying to communicate with the ambulance crew. They would just shrug their shoulders and go on talking to each other in French.

After what seemed like hours, but was probably only 10 minutes, a light grey passenger car pulled up in the lane next to ours. Two new attendants, dressed in different-colored attire, got out and walked slowly up to the ambulance. After greeting the original crew profusely, they exchanged places and we again proceeded down the highway. We later learned that we had reached some invisible political boundary and the original crew was not allowed to drive past that point. Unbelievable! We finally reached the little hospital in St-Pie. Mears was somewhat coherent by this time and asked why his car owner and I were staring at him.

We were greeted at the emergency room door by a big, ape-like, French-Canadian doctor. He sported a thick, bushy beard and was clad in Levis and an old flannel shirt. He carried a big knife on his belt. Even though it was the middle of summer, I was certain he had arrived by dog sled. He gruffly informed us that he was the only doctor on duty and he didn't have much time to spend. He also proclaimed proudly that he had just returned from a big trauma course at the university in Montreal, so this case was: 'no big deal'.

Following that announcement he proceeded to insert a urinary catheter into Mear's bladder, totally ignoring the fact that he was lapsing back into unconsciousness. I politely asked if there was a neurosurgeon on the staff.

"Are you kidding!" was the reply.

I grabbed Penske and told him we needed a helicopter immediately because his driver could have a significant head injury and we were in the wrong place. Penske went into action and acquired a helicopter, of sorts, within 20 minutes. Since the hospital had no landing zone, the chopper would need to land in the baseball field located across the street.

While the local doctor was still going through his assessment, Roger and I loaded Mears on to a rickety wooden cart with big wheels and walked him the 50 or so yards across the street to the landing zone. Soon, a helicopter emerged from the dank gloom that enshrouded the little town. As I guessed, it was not a true medical helicopter. It belonged to the Forest Service, the kind with the open sides you see in Vietnam movies.

Looking inside, I realized the floor was wooden. There were no seats, and the pilot was another French-Canadian who spoke no English. Seated ominously in a wooden box next to the pilot's seat were two open cans of motor oil. I could hardly wait.

As Penske and I loaded Mears on to the wood floor, the pilot grinned and poured one of the cans of oil into the engine. I hung the IV bag on to a nail in the ceiling while my patient continued to sleep peacefully. Fully awake, I was not so lucky. This was not fun! I hate helicopters. I had always been told to stay out of them. In my opinion, this was not a real helicopter at all. I reluctantly jumped inside as the pilot took off fearlessly for Montreal. Then I prayed.

After flying for about 20 minutes, without warning we nosed downward into a fairly rapid descent. I peeked down and, to my dismay, saw nothing but large pine trees. The pilot looked at me and grinned again. We continued to descend into what looked like certain death. Just when I thought we were going to crash, the trees seemed to part, revealing a narrow path to the ground below. The pilot was obviously a good one as the path through the pines was only a bit wider than the circling blades of our trusty aircraft.

We touched down softly on a bed of pine needles, landing in a small clearing just outside the trauma center of St. Mary's Hospital in Montreal. By this time, Mears' feet had ballooned to twice their normal size in spite of my having encased them in ice. He remained unconscious. Thankfully, a real trauma team met us at the door. They surrounded Mears and immediately went to work. My worst fear was that an enlarging blood clot might have formed over his brain similar to what Foyt had experienced in Michigan. It's not a good sign when you wake up and then go back into a coma following a blow to the head. I was relieved when his CT scan read as normal.

Attention was then focused back on to his ever-enlarging feet. They were discolored deeply purple and the pulses in both legs had disappeared. This meant that there was little if any blood reaching his feet. It would not take long for the tissue to begin to die. X-rays revealed multiple fractures. In fact, every bone in his right foot had been broken, all 27 of them.

The trauma team discussed the case at length and informed Penske, who had just arrived by car, and me that they would need to amputate. In defense of the Canadian way of doing things, this approach seemed economically sound. It was expedient and cost effective in that Mears could be up and around within a few months with prostheses. It was not, however, conducive to driving racecars, Mears' preferred occupation. Penske looked at me and I looked at him.

"Don't sign anything!" I said.

Mears' girlfriend Chris arrived about this time; I told her what was going on. Rather than panic, as many race drivers' girlfriends do, she calmly turned toward the nurses and asked what she could do to help. The hospital was chronically short staffed so the nurses allowed Chris to perform basic nursing duties. She also helped console Penske, who was still in sixth gear. He asked me what we should do now after refusing the Canadian doctors. I told him about Dr. Trammell in Indianapolis. I told him about Terry's success with Danny Ongais and that I thought he was as good as they get. I told Penske we needed to get Rick to Montreal as soon as possible for a second opinion. He told me to call Terry and immediately ordered one of his Learjets into the air. The locals thought we were all crazy. Mears slowly started to wake up. Chris remained remarkably calm.

I grabbed a phone and luckily got hold of Terry right away, often not an easy task. I told him he had to go to the airport because Penske's plane was going to land in 90 minutes and his future might depend on it. He told me he was on call at Methodist and there was no way he could do it. I reiterated that it was Roger Penske and surely he could figure something out. He said he would call back in a few minutes. Twenty minutes later he called back and said that he had coerced a partner into covering for him for one day only. He would have to be back the following morning to resume taking call. Terry had also called his wife who in retrospect, I think, was highly suspicious of his motives. The Penske jet was already within an hour of Indianapolis.

Trammell arrived at the Montreal hospital within three hours, courtesy of Penske Air. After viewing the X-rays and examining the patient, he agreed that the feet did not need to come off, at least not yet. Several small, deep cuts, called fasciotomies, had been made through the skin and underlying tissue to relieve the increased pressure that was impeding blood flow. Once the pressure was relieved, the blood vessels could re-expand, allowing blood again to flow into Mears' feet. He could safely remain in Montreal until after the race. The time spent in Montreal would allow the swelling in his feet to subside and assure me that no other occult injuries were liable to pop up.

Chris stayed at Rick's bedside assisting the nursing staff while Terry, Penske, and I met to formulate a plan to get him safely back to Indianapolis. Penske offered his air force in whatever capacity we thought might be helpful. I had to be back at the race track the following morning for practice and Terry had to return to Indy to keep his job. It was decided that Mears would stay in the hospital until Monday morning, Terry would return to Indy in the Learjet, and I would go back to the race track in the helicopter.

As we headed back to the ER, Terry pointed out that Mears would need a nurse to accompany him on Monday in order to administer pain medication and oversee his transfer and general wellbeing. He asked me if I knew an attractive brunette he had met while working at the Speedway in May. He thought her name was Lynne. He said she seemed like an excellent nurse who would do a capable job. What he didn't know was that I was seeing Lynne on the side. My second marriage was rapidly coming to an end and Lynne and I were having quite the steamy affair. I told Terry I would try to find her.

I located Lynne around 11:30 that night. When I finally made contact she was well oiled, carousing with some of her friends at the local drive-in. I informed her that she had to be at the airport by 7:00 am to meet Roger Penske's airplane. I relayed the whole story, that Dr. Trammell was coming back, and that she would need to locate some morphine and syringes. She told me I was nuts and hung up. I called her back and told her it was no joke and to get moving.

Lynne went to Methodist as soon as the movie was over and managed somehow to sneak the narcotics out of the hospital. She slept a couple of hours, awoke very early, and headed for the airport with a little brown bag full of morphine and syringes. She was sitting sleepily on the wooden bench just outside the aviation center when the Learjet landed.

Penske's pilots taxied the plane right up to the bench. Terry got out, and my girlfriend got in. Trammell gave Lynne a brief report on Mears and left hurriedly for his rounds at Methodist. Lynne flew off with the two pilots, a small suitcase, and the brown paper bag. Terry made it back to Methodist in time to take call and save his job.

The jet landed in Montreal two hours later. Onlookers would later describe a mysterious and beautiful Italian who had arrived by private jet, and then boarded a waiting helicopter whose engine had been kept running in anticipation. She was reportedly carrying a little brown paper bag and no one saw her go anywhere near the customs house.

The door closed on the mysterious passenger and the chopper disappeared into the late morning sky. Needless to say Penske is very well connected in Canada. Meanwhile, back at the race track, Edwards and I were sitting at our station as usual. A chopper approached shortly after the start of the morning practice period. It appeared from over the rim of an adjacent hill. Edwards pointed it out to me and said that it belonged to Penske. I looked at him with a straight face and said flatly:

"I know, he's bringing my girlfriend in for the race."

"Yeah, you wish," he said.

Edwards was in a state of serious shock when Lynne stuck her head through his window 10 minutes later. Penske had also arranged for a room in Montreal, and ferried Lynne and I back and forth to the track each morning in his helicopter. It was quite a weekend.

Mears remained stable, and on Monday morning Lynne and Chris flew with him back to Indy in the jet as planned. Before leaving the hospital they needed to find some pillows to elevate Rick's feet during the trip. Hospitals have a lot of pillows. In order to get four or five of them out of there the two women stuffed them under their clothes, feigning pregnancy as they left the building.

To avoid the media, who were camped in anticipation outside Methodist's emergency room, Lynne and Chris hustled the famous patient into the hospital through a little-known back entrance. Lynne and I had discovered it weeks earlier for surreptitious returns from the hotel across the street. The press was stymied and Mears went into surgery unhindered.

Dr. Trammell was waiting in the operating room and did a beautiful job repairing Rick's pulverized feet. He used previously developed hand surgery techniques on the feet for the first time. He was able to save both of them! Mears would require many other operations to complete the job, but this first surgery set the stage for a near full recovery.

Rick had to spend several months in the hospital recuperating from the extensive surgery, but he would eventually walk unassisted and most importantly, he would again drive racecars. He would later go on to win *two* more Indy 500s, in 1988 and 1991, as well as another CART Championship. Terry's reputation as a reconstructive orthopedist blossomed. Mears would eventually announce his retirement from racing in December of 1992, eight years after the accident. He was still competitive at the time of the announcement; he had simply lost his desire to compete after another near fatal crash that May during practice for the '500'. He is still acknowledged as the greatest oval track driver of all time.

As a result of the Mears' crash, and the number of orthopedic injuries we were experiencing in general, Penske and I began to lobby hard for CART to add an orthopedic surgeon to its traveling staff. We of course wanted Dr. Trammell to be that surgeon. CART, not wanting to add any more people to its roster, initially balked at the idea. To get around their reluctance, Penske began taking Terry to the races as his guest. One of these was CART's newest event, run in the parking lot of Caesar's Palace in Las Vegas. Roger set Trammell up in a luxury suit at Caesar's. With the rest of the CART officials, I was housed at the Hilton across the street.

Bad for him, but lucky for us, one of the support series drivers injured his back in a crash. Terry responded to the scene from his perch in the Penske pit and rendered the necessary orthopedic care. CART finally saw the light and allowed me to add Terry to the roster. He and I have been attending racing events together since that time in 1984.

As a direct result of the Mears crash, the dangerous steel barriers were finally banned forever from oval tracks. Additionally, the orthopedic component of our medical program was established, completing our ability to deal effectively with massive trauma.

Chapter 13

AL UNSER JR. AND CHIP GANASSI GET TOGETHER AT MICHIGAN

In 1984, CART once again gathered for the annual crashfest at the Michigan 500. Unusual for July, the day dawned grey and overcast. No rain was forecast, but the atmosphere encouraged a foreboding mood. Toward the midway point of the race the all too familiar call of 'Yellow! Yellow! Yellow' came through our radios. Here we go again. I was riding as usual with Steve Edwards in CART 1. We erupted from our station at the exit of Turn 1 and raced to a crash reported on the radio to be 'heavy' and 'bad'.

As we came out of the second turn, we could see what looked like two cars plastered against the inside wall about halfway down the back stretch. I had to admit it did look really bad. We turned into the infield grass and slid to a stop just in front of the worst-looking car. Chip Ganassi was slumped over unconscious in his totally destroyed racer. When I leaned into the cockpit, I thought he was dead. His eyes were dilated and his pupils did not appear to react. He wasn't breathing, he wasn't moving at all. The fact was, he appeared clinically brain dead.

Edwards and I secured his airway and began to do CPR. Thank God, he soon began to breathe on his own and his pupils dropped in size. We placed him in the ambulance and I rode with him to the helicopter already spooling up next to the track's infield care center. I met his father eye-to-eye as I stepped from the ambulance. Trembling, he asked me how his son was. I told him he was injured severely. I told him it didn't look good at all. Deep down, I didn't give Chip much of a chance.

Ganassi surprisingly woke up 10 days later. He was goofy, but able to respond to simple commands. Within a few weeks he was up and around and able to go home. I was very concerned that he would be permanently impaired. Later that same year, he showed up at a race and was obviously not the same old Chip. He would tell you a joke and then repeat it to you a few minutes later. The medical term that described Chip's new personality is hebephrenic, used to describe a person who was abnormally jovial and inappropriately unconcerned. He seemed totally unconcerned with reality and inappropriately happy, almost like he had had a few too many drinks. Everyone in the paddock thought Chip would never drive again or, for that matter, be able to hold down any kind of responsible position.

Within two years, however, he returned to normal in every respect. Today he owns one of the largest racing enterprises in the United States. He has a two-car team in the Indy Racing League, a three-car team in NASCAR, and a GrandAm team also with two cars. He is a principal player in NASCAR and owns part of the Pittsburgh Pirates baseball team. He is a multimillionaire and flies about the world in his private jet. His recovery from what appeared to be a devastating head injury was nothing short of miraculous. Why did Chip recover and so many other drivers in other series with similar injuries do so poorly?

We now know that much of the damage seen in head-injured patients is the result of a lack of adequate oxygen immediately following the injury. This lack of oxygen is often coupled with a significant drop in the blood pressure. The combination of lack of oxygen (hypoxia) with an inadequate blood pressure (hypotension) is catastrophic for full recovery. With the rapid response capabilities available in CART and at the Indianapolis Motor Speedway (USAC), injured drivers are not allowed to go without adequate oxygen for more than a few seconds and their blood pressure is supported immediately. The brain has an amazing ability to recover from a serious impact if secondary injuries are not allowed to occur because of a lack of timely response.

The seemingly phenomenal recoveries made by Indycar

drivers following potentially fatal head injuries is a direct result of the careful placement of the Safety Trucks and the combined expertise of the Safety Team. Medics on the street are not afforded this luxury because the crashes they attend have usually occurred several minutes or even hours before they can arrive. As a result, individuals who survive highway crashes usually do not recover neurologically nearly as well as do the racecar drivers.

Chapter 14

DALY DOES MICHIGAN

D r. Trammell and I continued to collect our crash and injury data as the 1984 season progressed and worked diligently to improve the safety of the CART series. One problem continued to hamper our efforts. It was very difficult at times to guarantee good equipment, personnel, and facilities at selected events. We still could not always rely on the promoters to provide the level of medical support we needed. Improperly equipped and poorly manned ambulances remained a frequent annoyance. Sometimes the ambulances were nothing but empty vans driven by track employees who were not at all versed in emergency trauma care. Left unchecked, promoters would often try to get away with whatever they could in order to fatten their bottom lines.

Infield care centers, when present, were still often inappropriately staffed and poorly equipped, serving more as a hospitality center for the local doctors and nurses than a proper emergency station. At the track in Riverside, California, for example, the track hospital was nothing but a wooden lean-to with a dirt floor. It looked like a tool shed. The medical director there appeared to be a barely functional alcoholic who was normally intoxicated before noon.

I complained incessantly about these things but it was very difficult in those days to get the promoters to spend money on medical and safety issues, and the CART sanction agreements didn't have the necessary teeth. Most of the promoters felt that since other racing organizations weren't so picky, CART didn't need to be either. We seemed to be fighting a continual uphill battle. Michigan International Speedway, however, was an exception.

The medical set-up there resembled the one at Indy. There was a properly equipped and staffed care center and the ambulance and helicopter services were exemplary.

Not long after the Mears crash in Canada, Derek Daly had a huge crash at MIS. He lost control of his car between Turns 3 and 4 during the Michigan 200 held in the Fall. He was traveling over 200 mph at the time. His car virtually disintegrated on impact, leaving both of his legs badly injured and totally exposed to the elements. Both were sticking morbidly out of the front of the tub. He bounced off the wall, spun 360 degrees, and continued sliding toward the wall for a second frontal impact still going over 160 mph with his legs leading the way.

A second impact would certainly have killed him because there was no protection left in the car. John Paul Jr., who was running behind Daly at the time, graciously T-boned him before he could hit the wall again. This second impact undoubtedly saved Daly's life. He suffered a fractured pelvis as a result of the impact with Paul, but miraculously never lost consciousness. The initial impact had fractured both of his ankles severely.

When Terry and I arrived at the scene, Daly was an easy extrication. All we had to do was unfasten his seatbelts and gingerly lift him from the car. The front of it was totally gone. His only comment to us at the time was that he was thirsty. He asked for water and began to describe the crash in vivid detail. He was perfectly lucid and remarkably calm. This calm demeanor following a near fatal accident is common in truly professional drivers. Rarely is their blood pressure the slightest bit elevated or their heart rate significantly altered after a really bad crash.

In fact, Pancho Carter had a huge crash while practising for the 1987 Indy 500 and exhibited a startling level of composure throughout the incident. He lost control of his car exiting the third turn at the Speedway, spun backwards, became airborne and actually flew upside down for several yards. When he landed on his head he was still traveling at well over 100 mph. Sliding on the pavement, he soon ground most of his rollover bar away. This left his helmet in contact with the asphalt. Carter phenomenally had the presence of mind to rotate his head to a new location, as soon as he felt the heat build up on his scalp due to friction as the track ground his helmet away. When I arrived at the scene, he had already extricated himself from the car, and took pride in showing me his helmet with three paper-thin circles as a testament to his clear thinking. Amateur drivers often do not show this professional demeanor following a crash.

Daly was airlifted to Ann Arbor, and the Michigan University Hospital, before I could intervene with the flight crew to tell them to go somewhere else. True to form, the Michigan staff would not allow Trammell or me to enter their intensive care unit. They would not even allow us phone access to Daly. They refused to meet with us at all, leaving us angrily standing in the hospital's main entrance. We learned what the doctors were planning only after talking to Daly's wife Beth on the hospital phone. She informed us they were taking him to surgery to fuse his fractured ankles. Terry became irate. Fusing the ankles would make them virtually useless for driving racecars. For that matter, it would eliminate him from any serious participation in most sports. We were helpless to intervene.

Daly was dragged off to surgery later that night and both ankles were fused. He remained in the hospital for several days following the surgery, growing progressively more depressed. He and his wife would call me almost daily to complain about the Michigan medical staff and the care they were giving. On one such call, Beth mentioned to me that the doctors appeared worried about a low red blood cell count. According to her, they kept transfusing him but they didn't run any tests to identify the source of the blood loss. They seemed satisfied just to keep giving him blood.

After receiving three calls in one night, I finally told Beth to sign her husband out of the hospital against medical advice and come back to Indianapolis. Advising drivers to sign out against medical advice was happening more often. Most physicians still viewed race drivers as uneducated daredevils bent on self-destruction.

When Derek arrived in Indy, Terry immediately took him back to surgery. He undid the work done in Michigan, giving him working ankles and a much better future as a driver. I obtained a CT scan of Derek's pelvis and found the source of his mysterious blood loss. He had fractured it in three places. Pelvic fractures are notorious for being difficult to discover and for continuously oozing blood over several days.

Daly's stay at Methodist Hospital happened to overlap that of Rick Mears, still recuperating from his crash in Canada. The two drivers were placed on the same floor of the hospital. Not a good idea. As a result, they soon terrorized the floor by racing their wheelchairs around the nursing station. This was good for their morale, but bad for the nurses. They were so competitive that even beating the other one out of the hospital became a challenge. Crashing often, they would sometimes jeopardize the hospital's physicians who were trying to make rounds. Most of the nursing staff, and many of the physicians, were very happy the day Mears and Daly finally left the hospital.

Death, fortunately, continued to leave CART alone and for that we were very grateful. Promoters continued to cut corners and we could not safely rely on them to provide the necessary emergency equipment. I longed for our own vehicle that could be available at every race supplied with all of the equipment we would ever need. A vehicle equipped well enough to carry out major life-saving efforts and to do minor procedures, and large enough to allow for private consultations and give us a place to hang our hats. Really wishful thinking!

Chapter 15

CART FULFILLS THE WISH

During the Mid-Ohio race in 1984, Jon Potter was approached by a man named Carl Horton. Horton owned the Horton Ambulance Company in Columbus, Ohio and was one of the most respected ambulance builders in the world. He was an affable guy who instantly hit it off with Jon. The two of them talked for most of the afternoon. Their discussion eventually turned to track safety issues and Horton told Potter that he had been trying unsuccessfully to get involved with the American Motorcycle Association. For some reason they had turned him down. He was now looking for another racing organization that could benefit from his company's involvement.

Horton told Potter about a pit incident he had seen on television that occurred during the 1981 Michigan 500. A huge fire had engulfed driver Herm Johnson's pit after a fuel fitting failed during the refueling process. This failure caused the entire pit to erupt in flames. Horton had watched the resulting chaos on TV and marveled at the way the CART Safety Team handled the very dangerous situation. He loved being around racecars as well as motorcycles and he was eager to play any kind of role he could. He thought the Safety Team might be a good vehicle to promote his company.

Potter introduced me to Horton that same day. He described him as the man sent to deliver us from the dark ages and into a new era of motorsports safety. In other words, Horton was the answer to my prayers. He had the money, the interest and the organization to get the job done. Jon and I arranged to see him later that Fall at his plant in Columbus, Ohio.

At the end of the season, we flew there on a cold, gloomy day in early November. We wanted to see the Horton factory in person and hopefully put a deal together for him to build a specialized rescue vehicle for the CART series. We flew in the private plane owned jointly by me and two of my friends. It was a turbocharged, twin-engined Beechcraft Duke previously owned by Winthrop Rockefeller. It had all of the necessary safety equipment and was well endowed with creature comforts. Tom Kirby, one of the owners and probably my closest friend, was the pilot. I had no business owning any part of an airplane due to my irrational fear of flying, but I was envious of the car owners who all did, and it was a convenient way to get to most of our races. Splitting the cost three ways made it just about doable.

I was a nervous flyer no matter what kind of plane I was in and did everything I could to stay on the ground. When we left the Indianapolis airport for Columbus, it was windy, dismally gray, and cold. Freezing rain was forecast. It was drizzling lightly when we took off and visibility was less than 500 feet. The day was much like the day Glenn Miller left for France during World War II.

I had boarded the plane reluctantly, and was not talking to anyone. I took my seat and quietly stared at the seatbelt sign. Sure enough, soon after takeoff, we encountered ice! This to me meant sudden death in a small plane. Kirby remarked calmly:

"Never fear, we have de-icing gear."

By this time, both wings and the tail had developed a thin sheet of ice. We were rapidly slowing down. I figured it was all over when Tom pushed the de-icing button and, like magic, the ice popped off the wings and tail. To my amazement and delight we were still flying!

As we began our descent into the Columbus airport my heart rate hit a new high. We were suddenly faced with severe crosswinds. It was all Kirby could do to land the plane. Once safely on the ground, he said he would wait for Jon and me until the meeting with Horton was over. In unison, we told him no thanks and to go on back to Indy without us. Just as we finished our remarks, a severe wind gust swept over the airport, nearly knocking me off my feet. At over 300 pounds, nothing could knock Potter off his feet. Kirby waved goodbye and taxied on to the runway. I truly never expected to see him alive again.

Jon and I rented a car and drove to Horton's company. During our meeting we discovered that he was the largest custom ambulance builder in the country. His operation was very impressive. The factory was neat, clean, and the employees all seemed proud and interested in what they were building. Following our tour, we went to Horton's office where we worked out a plan to develop CART's own special ambulance. It would be specifically equipped for race track medicine. Our ambulance would contain all the orthopedic supplies Terry would need and all the life support gizmos I would need. CART would provide a driver to take it to all the races. That evening, to seal our deal with Horton, we headed for the Columbus Country Club.

The club was Horton's favorite and frequent haunt. We headed straight for the bar. By midnight, Horton and I had each consumed in the neighborhood of seven Manhattans. As we progressed into the morning hours, the bartender politely asked us to leave. We had been the only ones left in the bar for some time. Potter and I reluctantly got into our rental car for the three-hour drive back to Indianapolis. It was 3:00 in the morning! Luckily, Jon had started drinking Coca-Cola early in the evening and was fairly sober. He became the designated driver. I felt miserable by then but was happy and, unfortunately, due in the hospital at seven o'clock that morning to make rounds. CART worked out the financial part of the deal with Horton and we anxiously awaited the next season and our very own medical unit.

Over the winter, Horton had invited Lynne and me to join him in Daytona Beach for their infamous Bike Week. He wanted us to share the experience. Horton's entourage stayed at the Holiday Inn right on the beach. I had never seen so many motorcycles gathered in one place. Every make, model, and type of motorcycle was represented. People and motorcycles took up every inch of available space.

Our first night in town we decided to visit the famous Boot Hill Saloon to celebrate our new partnership and the invention of the motorcycle. While waiting in line for a table, we overheard one biker chick ask her mate if he could find some salt for her beer. Wishing to please her, he promptly unzipped his pants and took a leak in her glass. She consumed the entire drink in one prolonged swallow and promptly asked for another one. Lynne and I couldn't believe it! Horton and his other guests were veterans of Bike Week, and hardly took notice.

Restrooms were at a premium in Daytona during Bike Week and I couldn't wait for the long line at the loo after dinner. It was an emergency! I went behind the saloon and carefully selected an area of the lawn furthest away from the crowd. Busily watering the grass, I was suddenly caught helplessly in the beam of the police helicopter's searchlight. The helicopter cop shouted something through his megaphone but I couldn't understand what he said. I soon realized that people had appeared all around me, waving and cheering me on. Lynne was extremely embarrassed. Horton loved it. He could be a lot of fun in those days.

Our new medical unit was completed late that winter just after our Daytona trip. Terry and I had constant input during the project, working closely with Horton's people. We were in heaven as we finally had a base of operations, a bit of privacy when seeing patients, and were assured of having the necessary equipment at our disposal. CART thanked Horton by naming the safety team after him. The Horton Safety Team, the only team like it in the world, began operations in the spring of 1985.

The Horton Safety Team soon developed into a highly skilled group of professionals. We became multi-faceted learning the intricacies of safely extricating an injured driver and quickly restoring a race track to its pre-crash configuration. The physicians on track would not only provide emergency medical care, they would also sweep up oil dry, pick up debris, direct traffic, and occasionally drive the Safety Truck. The Safety Team soon became the envy of racing organizations worldwide. Credit goes to the CART Board of Directors who, without hesitation, placed safety as their first priority and who, thankfully, appropriated the large sum of money it took to do the job. Well over $800,000 was needed annually to support the medical and safety programs.

Our first unit was the same size as a traditional box-style ambulance. We had reconfigured the lighting to provide brighter and more usable illumination. We added some basic orthopedic supplies such as splints, cast materials, and bandages. We upgraded the monitoring capabilities and expanded the available fluids and medications for advanced life support. The airway kit was also expanded. We would no longer have to rely solely on the track ambulances for proper resuscitation equipment.

Carl Horton really did love to have a good time. He and his wife Judy managed to attend nearly all of our races. The first race for the new Safety Team was Long Beach, California in April of 1985. At the time, it was considered the most beautiful venue on the CART circuit. The Long Beach Grand Prix was initially sanctioned by Formula One. That became too expensive so Chris Pook, the promoter and innovator of street racing in America, made a deal with CART to take over the race from 1984 onwards.

The backdrop for the 'Roar by the Shore' as the race was called, was the stately and picturesque *Queen Mary* docked forever in the Port of Long Beach. Lynne and I, Jon Potter, and Horton and Judy all went to dinner Friday night at Sir Winston's, an excellent restaurant on board the ship. It is still one of my favorites. Eating at Sir Winston's, with the sea on one side, and the coast of California on the other, actually made you feel like you were on a cruise. Most of the ship's amenities were still in their original condition, with the rooms modernized somewhat to fit the taste of the modern traveler.

After a large and sumptuous dinner, we retired to the lounge for some more drinks. The atmosphere was so perfect you would swear that Churchill himself was sitting at the bar. The lounge was also dead that night! The only things moving were the aged bartender, the humped-over, skinny little waitress, and a lonely couple whose marriage looked like it had ended some time ago. Elevator music had nearly bored everyone to sleep.

The five of us were about to leave when I spotted a dust-covered Steinway baby grand piano adorning a corner of the room. I pointed it out to Jon who was not seeing things too clearly by that time. We urged him to sit down and play. Jon didn't need much urging at that point as he staggered to the keyboard and began to pound out a little Jerry Lee Lewis. One song followed another and soon people began to traipse in from all over the ship. Within minutes, the place was packed and really alive. The bartender made more in tips that night than he had in a month. He begged us to stay. He asked repeatedly:

"Who is that guy?"

The bartender offered Jon a job right then and there. Jon played on until his fingers were ready to fall off. We reluctantly left a wildly cheering audience, as well as a very disappointed bartender, when someone pointed out that it was after midnight. Each of us had some serious work to do the next morning.

After leaving Sir Winston's, we foolishly decided to take a walk on deck to get some fresh air before going to bed. Feeling no pain at that point, we made our way to the top deck. We were admiring the stunning view of Long Beach when Potter remarked about how majestic the three smokestacks looked, each with a ladder going to the top. As a kid, I was really into climbing and the smokestacks were irresistible. So up I went.

Climbing the wire-like, dew-covered steps was quite a challenge. I nearly slipped on a couple of occasions, but managed to make it to the top. Once there, I grabbed the big searchlight and began to shine it back and forth over downtown Long Beach. This turned out to be a bad idea. While I was scanning the downtown, several police cars, with sirens screaming, arrived in the parking lot below. I was in deep shit!

I carefully climbed down while Potter began his elaborate

and articulate explanation as to why I was up there in the first place. Jon is a remarkable bull-shitter, but this was a lot to ask. Unbelievably, he convinced the local constables that I would never do it again, that no one had been hurt, and that he personally would see that I was put to bed. He also gave them some CDA pins and a few CART hats. They bought it! We went to bed straight away.

After-hour activities varied widely on the CART circuit in those days, and they were a lot more risqué than they are now. Scrutiny by the media, as well as the fear of lawsuits, makes life on the road much more sedate than it used to be. Maybe it's just that we've all grown up a lot more. For sure, everything is much more controlled and businesslike than it was in the 80s. The Long Beach Grand Prix began bright and early the next morning and the Horton Safety Team shone, although the doctor was a bit worse for wear.

We had continued to race at Sanair Speedway after Rick's horrible crash in '84 so we found ourselves there again in 1986. Nothing much had changed. There wasn't a lot to do for entertainment in that part of Canada, but our Safety Team was very resourceful. In St-Pie, the guys came across a large, converted farm silo where, for a small fee, you could ride on a massive column of forced air and practice your skydiving technique. Of course, none of our group skydived, but that was no reason not to give it a try.

One of the race teams employed an attractive blonde at the time who lived in Indianapolis. She had become somewhat involved with one of our Safety Team members. She too was practicing her skydiving technique that Friday night along with three quarters of the Safety Team. Suddenly, while fully spreadeagled over the column of air, she drifted too close to the edge. Losing all support, she fell some 40 feet to the floor below, badly dislocating her right knee. Lucky she didn't kill herself.

It was around 11 o'clock when the accident happened. Her blood alcohol level was nowhere near normal. What to do? Dr. Trammell, as luck would have it, had also ventured into the silo that evening. Upon seeing her fall, Terry did the most rational thing he could think of considering his similar state of inebriation. He drove her to our medical unit, parked and locked, behind our hotel. Puzzled, he then called my room from the phone in the lobby.

"Steve! You've got to come down here. We've got a big problem!"

I wasn't sure *we* had a problem, but I got dressed and went downstairs to assist my friend and colleague. The patient was not in too much pain when I arrived, largely due to the previously consumed alcohol. This was good. Her leg, however, was bent the wrong way at more than a 45-degree angle. That was bad.

Terry and his conscripted assistant spent the next hour or so reducing the severe dislocation at one o'clock in the morning, in our little ambulance, in the parking lot of the St-Pie Holiday Inn. Not exactly the approved standard of care at the time, but it did keep the incident relatively quiet. Our patient was able to keep her job with the race team and the incident went largely undetected.

We confined her to her hotel room for the rest of the weekend while our Safety Team member paid regular nursing visits. She flew with Terry and I back to Indy in the Methodist Hospital plane after the race. Her leg healed beautifully.

Our first Horton-designed specialized ambulance served us well for three years. It was driven to all the races by a delightful retired couple, Ned and Anne Miller. Soon, however, Terry and I realized we needed a bigger unit in order to do the things we felt we could get away with at the race track. We found we needed more headroom to allow us to do minor surgical procedures more comfortably. We needed room for more supplies, as well as the ability to tend to more than one patient at a time. The number of patients turning up at the medical center was increasing rapidly. We were treating crewmembers, media representatives, officials, owners, their families, and rarely drivers. Drivers actually comprised the fewest number of visits to the medical unit. If a driver showed up, he was usually really sick. Basically, we had created a monster. I don't think any other series or sports organization in the world tried to provide complete on-site medical care to its participants, with the exception of perhaps the Olympics.

We took care of anything we thought we could get away with. Cold and 'flu patients were abundant. We also sewed up several lacerations that could easily have qualified as hospital-based surgical procedures. Terry cast, splinted, and reduced several orthopedic injuries. VD, foreign bodies in the eye, and even psychiatric counseling were all common occurrences. I treated a number of cardiac arrythmias (abnormal heart rhythms) and diagnosed a few heart attacks. We did 'home' dialysis on one official, and once gave an injection to actor Paul Newman.

Our tiny medical center was getting a real work out. We had simply outgrown it. Terry and I met with Horton at his factory at the end of the 1987 season to design a new model. He suggested using a fifth-wheel trailer as the basis for the new unit. This would provide the much-needed space and headroom and would be relatively easy for the Millers to drive around the country.

A rapid design process ensued and construction began that winter. In the spring, we were presented with a new unit four times as large as the original with a reception area and walk-in capabilities. We could now care for more than one person at a time. When the new unit went into service our admission rate grew even larger. I realized that a nurse was needed to handle the admission of patients, the increased paperwork, and to provide nursing assistance to Terry and me as we grew busier.

During any given race weekend, Terry and I would normally be stationed on the race track any time the cars were running. There would be no one minding the store in the medical unit. On one such occasion Jim Chapman, the head of PPG Racing, CART's major sponsor, developed a dangerously abnormal heart rhythm while entertaining prospective customers in his hospitality tent. He was rushed by friends to our medical unit for treatment. No one was there. The practice session that was in full swing had to be red flagged so I could be brought in to take care of Mr. Chapman. A nurse was definitely needed.

Terry and I suggested that Lynne be hired as the CART nurse. Many of the participants already knew her and she had done a great job during the Mears incident. The CART brass agreed, and hired her. She went to work immediately, maintaining the expanding supply and equipment list as well as providing emergency care when Terry and I were on track. He and I were actually becoming the 'family physicians' for most of the CART participants. Many of the crew guys and other support personnel were on the road three quarters of the year. Several were from out of the country. They did not have the time, or the ability to seek medical attention at home, so they sought it from us.

We followed patients with high blood pressure, diabetes, and even chronic kidney disease. We counseled husbands and wives and did damage control when necessary. We began to develop an intimate association with most of the families whose lives revolved around the CART series. Carla Carter even suggested a soap opera entitled 'As the Wheels Turn'. The organization was indebted to Carl Horton now more than ever.

Chapter 16

LIVES SAVED

D r. Trammell had become very busy with his private orthopedic practice in Indianapolis and it was impossible for him to attend all of the CART races. We needed another orthopedist to fill in when Terry had to be at work. Joe Randolf, one of Terry's partners, volunteered for the job. Now 'Gucci' Joe, as we called him because of his constant attention to sartorial splendor, was not your typical dyed-in-Nomex racing nut. When he was asked about the size of firesuit he would need, he politely stated that he didn't need one because he wasn't going to be near any fires. He was not planning to get too close to the cars either. He abhorred getting dirty and the thought of grease and oil on his designer clothes was unthinkable.

Joe would normally spend a race weekend in PPG's hospitality tent, a gathering place for the credentialed multitudes and VIPs. There, Joe would hang out with the pace car girls, shoot the breeze with major corporate types, and rub elbows with the frequent celebrity guests. On one of Joe's weekends, he found himself in the tent as usual talking to Jim Chapman during a practice session for the Milwaukee race. He was sipping an iced tea when suddenly an emergency call came through his radio.

"Dr. Randolf, you're needed in the Med Center Stat!"

Joe politely excused himself and made his way back to the medical center. An elderly local official had unfortunately collapsed in the pit area and was in full cardiac arrest. The incident had been observed by our two roaming paramedics who rushed to the scene and had already begun the initial resuscitation. They were soon *en route* to the medical unit with the patient on the MR-10. The MR-10 was another Horton design; a golf-cart of sorts, equipped with all of the emergency resuscitation essentials and a full-length stretcher for the patient, as well as fire-retardant chemicals and oil dry for use in the pits. I had recently added this new vehicle in order to cover the pit and paddock areas since a conventional ambulance would simply not fit in some of the tight confines and was especially difficult to maneuver through a large crowd. With two medics on the MR-10 in constant motion throughout the paddock and pit areas, we could rapidly respond to any emergency that might develop.

The MR-10 had luckily been stationed close to the man when he collapsed. Lynne and Joe waited anxiously for the patient in the new medical unit. If the man only knew what was in store for him. Reportedly, Joe's heart also nearly stopped when he was told what was coming. But, in perfect 'Gucci' form, he stood at the head of the bed nodding his approval at the way Jerry Guise and Lynne saved the man's life.

Joe went back to PPG after the rude interruption without a trace of blood or other bodily fluid anywhere on his new outfit. Joe was, and still is, a brilliant orthopedic surgeon. He has operated successfully on a number of racing personalities and other sports celebrities. He loved the ambiance that surrounded the track, but had no desire to deal in emergency medicine if he could avoid it. All kidding aside, Joe did help to save that old man's life. The patient who arrested that day went on to survive and was the first life actually saved in our new medical unit.

Later in the summer, we were racing again at the very fast Michigan International Speedway. Phil Krueger, a struggling driver at the time, crashed heavily during the event and was brought to the medical unit. He was accompanied by Dr. Crippen who had overseen the extrication. Krueger was unconscious and gasping for air when he arrived in the unit. Crippen and I rapidly diagnosed a collapsed lung caused from several broken ribs. It was not possible for him to breathe adequately without a tube being placed in his chest to re-expand the collapsed lung. He would also need a tube placed in his windpipe to protect his airway as he was in a deep coma, the result of a severe head injury. He had vomited a large amount and his face was a mess.

Crippen went to work on the chest tube while I began to place the tube in his trachea. It was a very difficult situation but we managed to get the tubes in the right places and a second life was saved in the unit. Krueger's head injury turned out to be a bad one, causing him to endure a long period of rehabilitation. He managed a return to racing for a short time, surprisingly driving better than he did before he crashed. He qualified for Indy in both 1986 and '88, something he hadn't been able to do before his injury. He remained active as a car owner following his retirement and would actually fly to the U.S. races in his own airplane.

Once again, Michigan International Speedway proved to be a volatile race track. Due to the large number of serious crashes that occurred there, I had expectantly added a third doctor to the team in Michigan. Trammell, Crippen, and I worked together there for several years. Crippen and Trammell were stationed in their respective trucks strategically positioned around the race track. I remained in the medical unit with the closed-circuit TV monitor and a communication command center. It proved to be a good set up as Krueger's accident definitely tested the system. With two doctors on track, me in the hospital, and the MR-10 in the pits we felt that we had our bases fairly well covered.

Chapter 17

PUSHING THE
MEDICAL ENVELOPE

In the fall of 1987, I was getting my hair cut on a beautiful sunny afternoon in Indianapolis. The hair salon was in the quaint little village of Broad Ripple located on the near north side of Indianapolis, several miles from the Speedway. Halfway through my haircut I received an emergency page on my beeper. The news wasn't good. Roberto Guerrero, Colombia's best driver at the time, had crashed heavily while testing tires for Goodyear at the Indianapolis Motor Speedway. Roberto had recently joined the CART series from Formula One, and was extremely fast, rising to the top of the sport very quickly. Medics from the scene reported a severe head injury with the patient in a deep coma. Guerrero was unable to breathe for himself and required assisted ventilation *en route* to Methodist Hospital.

I jumped from the barber's chair with only half a haircut and sped to the hospital. When I arrived at the emergency room, I was met by Dr. Bock who was on duty that day. Mike Turner, an excellent neuro-trauma surgeon, was on hand as well. They both reported that the head injury looked really bad. The CT scan of Guerrero's head did not reveal anything that the surgeons could fix. Sadly, it showed instead a very swollen brain with severe diffuse axonal injury, or DAI. Basically, the brain had suffered an extensive shearing injury to the nerve fibers causing the entire central nervous system to short circuit. It could not be surgically repaired. Guerrero was moved directly from the emergency room to the intensive care unit.

The cause of this injury in the general public is usually a motor vehicle accident. The forces of a crash, if severe enough, cause the head to violently rotate. Severe damage can occur to the brain without the head ever coming into contact with anything. Nerve fibers within the brain and brainstem are damaged by this shearing effect. A helmet offers virtually no protection for this type of injury. The mortality rate in the general population was reportedly over 80% in 1987. The only treatment was, and still is, supportive care. Judicious use of medications to help remove the excess brain water and to control the increased pressure that develops inside the skull are the only modalities of therapy.

One promising treatment had recently been tried in some large medical centers with varying degrees of success. It was not yet in common usage. Many neurologists and neurosurgeons did not feel it was beneficial and were reluctant to try it. The treatment involved the use of barbiturates in very high, even toxic, doses given intravenously. The medication was thought to decrease the metabolism of the brain and, as a result, lower the pressure inside the brain itself. If the brain was allowed to swell too much, it would herniate or rupture through the opening in the base of the skull called the foramen magnum. This extrusion of the brainstem would usually result in immediate brain death.

We had used barbiturates to treat increased brain swelling on a number of other occasions, but only in the standard recommended doses. We had never used the very high experi-mental doses that had been reported in the medical literature. Dr. Turner and I met with Guerrero's wife Kati and told her the gravity of the situation. We told her there wasn't anything to do surgically and that the only hope for her husband was supportive care and the use of the high dose barbiturate therapy. We asked for permission to use these very high doses. Kati grasped the situation fully and told us to do anything we thought might save her husband's life.

Dr. Turner and I placed him in an artificial coma with the barbiturates. He required the ventilator for breathing support and constant monitoring of his vital signs. A probe was placed inside his brain to measure his intracranial pressure. It was sky high!

Normal was less than 15, his was over 60! I started pushing the barbiturates intravenously. We reached the usual maximum dose with no effect on the pressure inside his head. The situation looked grim. I then gave five times the recommended dose. This caused his blood pressure to drop precipitously to near zero. I thought he was dying. I quickly started another medication to raise his blood pressure. He required huge amounts of this medicine. I was not at all hopeful. Kati remained at his bedside, determined.

After about seven hours of this treatment, and, after a lot of criticism including accusations of experimentation from the nursing staff, the pressure inside Guerrero's brain began to subside. Within 24 hours it was back to normal. He woke up three weeks later. I had spent most of the first 36 hours of his hospitalization at the bedside. His wife never left him at all! She remained by his side throughout his entire stay in the intensive care unit. She would later accompany him daily during his long rehabilitation process.

When Guerrero first spoke, he spoke in Spanish, his native language. He told Kati he loved her. He steadily progressed, and eventually was ready for a long and difficult rehabilitation. Spurred on by Kati and his young son Marco, he took his rehab to heart. He was one of the first patients to receive what we call cognitive rehabilitation. This form of rehab used computer-assisted exercises designed to bring a person's memory and visual motor skills back to baseline via biofeedback. It was very much like playing a series of complicated video games. Guerrero was scheduled to spend five hours a day doing these exercises. He would spend nine. During this period he would also relearn to walk and to speak the English language.

Kati was unrelenting, pushing hard. As a result of her efforts, her determination, and her deep affection, Guerrero was driving the family car within two months and actually played a full game of golf in three. His recovery surprised all of us.

In April of 1988, he wanted to drive a racecar again. His team entered him in the race at Phoenix. I thought he could do it as well because he appeared to me to be totally recovered. No one else seemed to think so. Due to justifiable apprehension on the part of the other CART officials, as well as his fellow drivers, I subjected him to a full nine-hour battery of neuro-psychiatric tests. He passed them all with flying colors! I repeated the tests for a second time at the University of California in Los Angeles (UCLA) medical center just to assure the officials that the tests were not biased. Again he passed! At UCLA, he was also continuously monitored for any seizure activity. He had none. He was then required to go through a strict driving test under the watchful eyes of CART Chief Steward Wally Dallenbach. Again he passed! CART had no choice but to clear him to race. I was as anxious as a whore in church.

Guerrero qualified second in the field of 28 cars. Some of the other drivers would barely speak to me. The only two people, other than Roberto, who were convinced he could drive, were Kati and me. Once the race started I could barely function. All I could think of was what if he crashed and hurt or killed someone else? I would never be forgiven in spite of the precautions I had taken.

After the start, Guerrero held on to second place. He began passing lapped cars as if possessed. He passed on the outside as well as on the inside. Phoenix is a one-mile oval track with each lap taking only 25 seconds. Negotiating heavy traffic on such a fast and tight course is what made the short ovals so spectacular to watch. Roberto was awesome! He would finish second that day less than six months after his devastating and usually fatal head injury. I was vindicated on all counts. Because of my experience with him, head injury became my primary focus of study. Guerrero went on to race for many more years. He and Kati are still married and live in California with their two boys. It is amazing what persistence, love, and dedication can accomplish. Also, a certain degree of really good luck!

Chapter 18

HORTON'S FALL
FROM GRACE

Lynne Olvey was working out great as the CART nurse. She had performed flawlessly during the Rick Mears incident and seemed the ideal choice for the Horton Safety Team. The drivers and crew guys loved her, and it made going to the races much more enjoyable for me. Unfortunately, this happy situation was not to continue. Lynne and I could not always go to the same races. Sometimes she was forced to go alone because I had to remain at home to take call at the hospital.

One of these occasions was a race at Mid-Ohio. Lynne planned to drive to the event with her four-year-old son Kyle. CART had a bad habit of putting their workers up in motels out in the middle of nowhere, often miles from the race track. Mid-Ohio was a perfect example. For this event, the chosen motel was located in a dismal little town called Bucyrus. A real hick town, Bucyrus was located more than 45 minutes from the track. To get to the track, you had to negotiate your way over and around several poorly marked country roads. Lynne got lost the first morning she was there and, as a consequence, was late for the weekend's first practice session.

Carl Horton had unfortunately picked that day to entertain some of his business associates from Columbus. He was hoping to give them a tour of the medical unit first thing that morning. He was waiting at the door when Lynne arrived. He confronted her angrily, berating her in front of his guests. Lynne, being Italian, gave it right back. Horton didn't like that at all and fired her on the spot. This was the nurse who made straight As in college, taught other nurses critical care, and took care of Rick Mears. I could not understand Horton's reaction. The only explanation I could imagine was that he wanted to get rid of me. He had to assume that I would be so angry I would resign. I almost did. But why would he want me to resign? One can only surmise that he wanted me out of there in order to move CART's base of medical and safety operations to his home town of Columbus, Ohio. He had recently hired Edwards to work full-time for his company, taking him away from the CART office in Michigan. Edwards had already made the move to Columbus and was beginning to centralize the Horton effort. Horton was a prominent figure in Columbus and on the Board of the local trauma center. It would be a definite feather in his cap to move the medical and safety operations there.

Terry Trammell, Wally Dallenbach, and Mario Andretti stood up for me when Horton tried to convince the CART Board that Lynne and I were not good for the organization. It became apparent to Horton that Terry and I were in the CART community to stay. To defuse the situation, Terry was made Director of Medical Services and dealt one-on-one with Horton. I continued as Director of Medical Affairs and dealt more with the local hospitals and the tracks. Our relationship with Horton was strained following the incident.

Around the time Lynne left CART we were in the process of designing a replacement unit for the fifth-wheel trailer. Our third unit was to be a vast improvement over the first two as it would be totally self-contained. It would be larger and even better equipped to withstand the rigors of the open road. We were continuously adding more equipment and supplies. This third unit, also built by Horton, was designed around a Greyhound bus chassis and when completed was as plush as any country singer's motorhome. The new unit went into service at the beginning of the 1989 season.

No medical team in the entire sports world had ever enjoyed anything like it. As we were expanding, so was the series, and so was the need to hire more personnel. With Lynne gone we needed two new nurses. Sue Dunham and Liz Deluca were both added to the team. Each of them had trained at Methodist and Lynne orientated them to the CART medical system. Sue had worked for several years in the emergency department and was well trained in acute trauma care. Liz worked in my intensive care unit as a critical care nurse and was an expert in critical care decision making and the care of complex patients.

We also added another physician, Jay Phelan. The race schedule now went from March through October and the races numbered more than 20. Jay was a Navy doctor who specialized in ear, nose, and throat surgery. He was also the flight physician for 'Top Gun', the Navy's fighter pilot training center in Miramar, California and no stranger to acute care medicine.

Soon after our newest unit was placed into service, the Horton Ambulance Company was forced into bankruptcy. Horton ended up selling the Safety Team back to CART. The circumstances of the bankruptcy were never divulged and we have not seen or heard from Horton since. From that time on, the Team was renamed the CART Safety Team and was under CART's total control with Edwards in charge of safety and Trammell and me taking care of medical issues.

Chapter 19

EMERSON ARRIVES

At the start of the 1985 season, a driver broke on to the CART scene making more of an impact than anyone else I could remember. He was arguably the most charismatic driver in CART's history. He was originally assigned to drive a pink car owned by a suspected drug dealer from Miami. The thought of a foreigner racing a pink car at Indianapolis made A.J. Foyt sick to his stomach. Foyt assumed all foreigners to be of questionable sexual orientation until proven otherwise and there was no chance any of them could drive a racecar as well as he could. He had conveniently forgotten about former World Champions Jimmy Clark, Jackie Stewart, Graham Hill, and several other European drivers who had raced successfully at Indy in the 60s.

Emerson Fittipaldi had twice been World Champion and was, without question, one of Formula One's greatest drivers. For 33 years he remained the youngest driver to have become World Champion, beating 1997 champion, Jacques Villeneuve, for that honor by only two months until Fernando Alonso finally took over the accolade in 2005.

Emerson's long, sweptback hairstyle and sideburns made him appear as unique and memorable as any rock star. Standing still he looked like he was going fast. He carried with him an entourage befitting royalty. His smile was irresistible, with the personality to match. He took the CART paddock by storm.

Fittipaldi had previously suffered a series of financial setbacks in Brazil after leaving Formula One as a driver. He had tried unsuccessfully to field his own Formula One team, working alongside brother Wilson. He was encouraged to return to racing by a good friend of mine, Ralph Sanchez. Sanchez was the creator of the very successful Miami Grand Prix and talked Fittipaldi into driving in the Miami street race in 1984. Emerson was nearly bankrupt at the time and gratefully accepted the offer. He didn't finish the race, going out with mechanical trouble, but he made a very credible showing after winning the pole position.

José 'Pepe' Romero was impressed with Emerson and asked him to be the driver for his newly formed Indycar team. The year-old March Fittipaldi would drive, if he accepted the deal, was painted a hideous pink color. The team Romero assembled to support Fittipaldi lacked both experience and ability. As a consequence, Emerson struggled during his first season in CART. Even so, he was still able to exhibit some periods of truly brilliant driving. He also continued to be very impressive off the race track due to his hugely marketable personality. Always demonstrating the promotional talents needed to succeed in the new world of business-driven motorsports, he caught the eye of several car owners.

Pat Patrick was one of them. Patrick soon negotiated a deal with him. In 1987, with good equipment, Emerson started to win races. He began to attract more and more media attention as the season progressed. Patrick Racing was soon forced to enlarge their hospitality area just to accommodate Emerson's expanding flock. He would bring his entire family to most of the events along with his cook, his masseuse, his trainer, his nutritionist, and his PR person. He flew all of them in the jet he purchased shortly after signing the deal with Patrick.

I must admit that I was also captivated by Emerson's arrival in CART. He was usually surrounded by beautiful women and seemed to know everybody connected with the sport. He had an aura about him not seen before in American racing. Not even A.J. Foyt, Rutherford, or the Unsers attracted the attention Emerson did. In addition to all the excitement surrounding his mere presence in the paddock, he talked with this really great accent. I made it a point to get to know him.

By 1987, I had developed a very close relationship with the Patrick race team. In fact, Pat Patrick had named me as a consultant to his petroleum company in 1983. In that capacity, I consulted on company medical issues, as well as provided medical care to Mr Patrick and his family. It was through Patrick Racing that I met Emerson.

I was asked by the team to attend a private test in Sebring, Florida in the winter of 1987. It was Emerson's first year with Patrick and he was getting familiar with the team and the new car. During the down times, when the mechanics were making adjustments or repairs to the car, there was absolutely nothing to do in Sebring. Emerson and I had plenty of time to get acquainted. We would sit somewhere in the sun and discuss cars, boats, planes, and our troubled marriages. Both were stormy at the time, and both involved stepchildren and the associated jealousies with the new wife.

We soon discovered that we had a lot in common. Even though our backgrounds were vastly different, and outwardly we were so dissimilar, our opinions about women, marriage, sports, politics, and life in general were much the same. We began a friendship that has lasted for nearly 20 years.

Until Emerson arrived on the scene, Indycar drivers were characterized as being brave and strong, but not necessarily fit. Most of them had honed their driving skills on the wild and dangerous midget and sprint car tracks scattered in small towns throughout America. Driving these cars on short ovals required a lot of manhandling but not necessarily a lot of finesse. The public all drove cars and that wasn't demanding at all. Most people assumed that driving a racecar wasn't any different; you just went faster and risked life and limb. The typical American racing driver at the time was thickly built and physically powerful, but not really fit in the athletic sense. The public, as well as most physicians, did not consider drivers to be athletes. They were never looked upon in the same way as football, baseball, and basketball players, or any of the other traditional athletes. Emerson changed this stereotype forever when he introduced the concept of true fitness to the American motorsports scene.

Competition in Europe by the 80s had become so intense that drivers were forced to be in peak physical condition to have any hope of being competitive. If a driver wasn't fit, he didn't get a job. Car handling had improved steadily over the years, resulting in a dramatic increase in the G loads experienced by the drivers. This increase in lateral Gs led to an increase in the physical input necessary to combat the loads. In a 5G corner a three-pound helmet suddenly weighed 15. The driver had to exert a huge amount of effort just to keep his body upright and in a proper driving position. Much greater upper body strength, flexibility, and endurance were needed. Aerobic training had quickly become a necessary part of the driver's daily routine. By 1980 most of the big teams in Europe had employed their own trainers, nutritionists, and massage therapists.

Emerson brought this whole scene to Indycar racing. He imported his cook from Brazil and his trainer, Gary Smith, from Aspen. Smith was a self-styled fitness guru who had convinced several other famous sports celebrities to work with him. He commanded a large fee. His mystic and intense Oriental training was reportedly acquired while serving in Vietnam during the war. He managed to gain Emerson's confidence while the Fittipaldis were on a skiing holiday in Colorado. Gary was charismatic, as well as knowledgeable, and Emerson adopted him into the entourage.

One afternoon while working at the hospital I received a call from Emerson.

"Steve, Gary would like you to be in a commercial for his new diet. He'll even pay you for it!"

Somewhat broke at the time, I excitedly agreed and met the film crew outside the hospital later that same day. By the time the film crew had set up their lights and cameras it was growing dark. I was hurriedly offered a contract that I signed even though I couldn't see the small print in the fading light. As a result, I gave away all rights to any royalties from the sale of the diets. I also allowed the company to use my likeness and image forever. Not smart!

The infomercial for the Aspen Wellness Diet ran for about four years in several countries. The diet consisted of a variety of soups made with all of the essential nutrients. If consumed as directed, the dieter could expect to lose up to eight pounds in only seven days. It was actually a good diet for athletes at the end of their off-season to shed unwanted pounds gained while not competing.

The product was a great success, eventually being sold in all of the Sharper Image and Walgreen stores. My picture ended up on the boxes right along with Emerson's. I received a one-off payment, while Emerson's royalties, I believe, continue to this day. He had read the small print and I learned a tough lesson.

The Aspen diet made a lot of money for both Emerson and Gary. Emerson trained hard during this period and ate what Gary told him to eat. His macrobiotic diet consisted of, among other things, kelp, weird fruits and humus. He also drank gallons of tiger milk. In my quest to be like Emerson, I instructed my wife to seek out the ingredients of a macrobiotic diet.

Lynne searched for, and finally found, a macrobiotic market in a remote and dangerous part of Indianapolis. She prepared the first macrobiotic meal at our home on a school night. Seaweed was the principle ingredient along with some other strange pieces of animal and vegetable matter. My 15-year-old daughter Dawn, and Lynne's son Kyle who was 12 at the time, sat down to eat with us. Lynne placed the dinner on the table. The kids bolted for the door.

"YUCK!"

I tried to stick with the diet for about a week and gave up. Emerson followed the diet religiously. Eating mostly things from the ocean, he thrived! We tested Emerson's fitness at the Performance Institute at Methodist Hospital in Indy and found him to be in a league of his own compared to the other American drivers. His cardiovascular fitness, strength, and endurance were that of an Olympic athlete. His reaction times matched those of a professional hockey goalie. He had only 13% body fat.

The days of the big, tough, musclebound driver were gone forever. Drivers in the upper echelon of motorsports today are all physically very fit as well as very lean. Excess body fat can cause a loss of concentration, not a good thing at 200 mph when you are traveling at more than a soccer pitch a second. Excessive weight also leads to temperature intolerance and a decrease in reaction times. Couple that with fatigue and you have a disaster in waiting. A driver simply can no longer be competitive or safe unless he or she is totally fit.

Competition, coupled with a general downsizing of the cockpit for aerodynamic reasons, has caused the average size of drivers to decrease steadily over the years. They now approach jockeys in height and weight. The average driver in Indy and Formula One cars is currently around five feet seven inches tall and weighs 148 lbs. Emerson was five feet eight and weighed in at 150 lbs. He continued to win that year for Patrick Racing.

Financially well heeled, Patrick Racing was able to do a lot of off-season testing. Individuals not intimately involved in racing do not realize that a race driver actually works year round. One of the places they liked to test was the track at Sebring, Florida because Sebring most closely duplicated a typical temporary road circuit.

During his first off season, following a day of testing a new car in Sebring, Emerson, along with his team manager, Jim McGee, his engineer, Morris Nunn, and I went into town for dinner. Sebring's population at the time consisted mostly of retired people who played golf while waiting patiently to die. Sleepy little southern town says it all. We picked out the only Italian restaurant for dinner. The average age in the place was easily mid-70s. The lounge smelled suspiciously of the American Association of Retired Persons (AARP).

While voraciously consuming our dinners, we were suddenly interrupted by a very pale and anxious-appearing maitre d'. In a feeble, shaking voice he told us that a bomb threat had just been made against the restaurant and he thought we should quickly leave. We hurriedly left the building. Jim, Morris, and I got as far as the front doorstep when we stopped our rush to leave and waited patiently to return to our table. We couldn't imagine any of the elderly citizens of Sebring setting off an explosive device, no matter how disgruntled they might be.

Emerson, we realized, was nowhere to be found. We looked in the parking lot, we looked behind the building, and we looked back inside, no Emerson!

"There he is!" shouted Jim. "He's across the street!"

The street he was on the other side of is six-lane Highway 27, no lonely country road. It dissects Sebring in the north and south directions. Speeding cars and trucks, desperately trying to escape the town, crowd the road at all hours of the day and night. When Emerson finally did make it back to the restaurant, he informed us, in a very serious tone of voice, that we were not from Brazil where bomb threats were taken quite seriously! We had a good laugh and went back in to eat. Testing was scheduled to resume the next day.

Emerson was such a good test driver that he could tell right away whether or not a car was any good. The Patrick team would wait anxiously every time a new car was delivered, hoping Emerson would be happy with it. If he didn't like it right away, then forget it. No amount of persuading would ever convince him to drive the car fast. This attitude infuriated Mo Nunn but Emerson was usually right.

In 1989 a new car was unloaded and it looked like a beauty. Emerson fell in love with it right away. He named this new Lola, 'Lolita'. Emerson and 'Lolita' were dominant throughout the entire '89 season, winning both the Indianapolis 500 and the CART Championship for Pat Patrick and his team. Emerson was now CART's premier driver. His intensity and his desire to win were unwavering.

The morning before the '89 '500' I met briefly with Emerson in his garage just before he left for the starting grid. Race morning in Indianapolis is special to all race fans. The air is electric, filled with excitement, apprehension, and great expectation. Hordes of people wander about the facility. As early as six o'clock in the morning many of them cram their faces against the garage area fencing, trying to catch a glimpse of their favorite driver. On this morning, Emerson was more focused than at any other time I could remember. The look on his face was a mixture of confidence and cruelty. His eyes bore through the masses as we left the garage. He simply said:

"Steve. I go to race now."

I knew he was going to win. In the future, whenever Emerson had that look, he would win. He was the consummate racing driver. His fitness schedule in Miami included two hours of Karate in the morning, two hours of running in the heat of the day at noon, and one hour of weight training in the evening. He was religious about it. He was probably in better shape than 98% of men half his age. His entire being was focused on winning. He did all of this while managing a vast array of businesses with holdings in five countries. He spoke five languages and became the most popular foreign driver ever to race in the U.S. I soon realized that I could not be like Emerson; not even close!

Chapter 20

THE GOOD YEARS
IN CART

CART was booming throughout the 80s and into the mid-90s. Crowds were massive and the racing was superb. We had not had a fatality since 1982 and severe injuries were on the decline. The foot and ankle injuries, so numerous in the 70s and early 80s, had basically disappeared thanks to our dogged record keeping and the subsequent design changes. During an average season, we had no more injuries than most professional football or hockey teams. Terry and I continued to keep accurate injury statistics and we were learning a lot about racecar safety and injury prevention. The two of us were giving talks on racing safety around the country, but we weren't sure if anyone was listening. In spite of our frequent speaking engagements, our data was still being largely ignored by the academic community. Most professors still regarded racing as a foolish endeavor and not a valid sport. In their opinion, race drivers were simply brave and crazy risk takers.

The Safety Team was evolving as well. Working races on the many road courses that now comprised most of the series, proved to be much more physically demanding than working just oval tracks. Australia, added to the schedule in 1991, introduced the consequences of jetlag to the CART community. No longer could a Safety Team member expect just to sit in the truck and munch on snacks for most of the day. He needed a reasonable level of fitness to survive the rigors of frequent travel and the demands of pushing and pulling errant racecars out of harm's way from various run-offs and tire barriers from circuit to circuit. Once, on a very hot day in Toronto, the temperature inside our truck was measured at over 130 degrees. We were in and out of that truck for eight straight hours. I consumed 12 standard-sized bottles of water during that day alone.

Steve Edwards was still our Safety Director but his days were numbered. A series of misadventures had caused Wally Dallenbach, and the rest of the senior officials, to question whether or not Edwards was the best man for the job. No one found fault with his abilities or his desire to do the job. In fact, he had a phenomenal ability to sort out quickly any variety of complicated situations. The problem with Edwards was his lack of tact with local safety personnel.

Narrow escapes from being run over by an oncoming racecar were becoming more frequent. He was frequently getting into disputes with the local safety providers and once went so far as to provoke a fist fight with the track's safety director during a green-light session in Phoenix. Coming into town with the medical and safety army we had acquired was not always met with favor by local personnel. A great deal of tact was now required in order to enable the two teams to mesh comfortably with each other. Dallenbach finally asked Edwards to resign his position as Safety Director and this happened in the summer of 1989. It was sad in many ways, but the sophistication of the sport now required a different type of personality.

Lon Bromley, one of the top medics on the Safety Team, was named Safety Director to replace him. Bromley brought a more tactful and logical approach to the job. He had been an employee of Dallenbach's in New Jersey and had followed the Dallenbach family to Colorado to help develop their ranch in Basalt. After moving to Colorado, Dallenbach discovered that there was no effective emergency medical care in and around the town of Basalt. He and his wife Pepe were bringing up two very active boys and one equally active girl. The entire family was outdoors most of the time doing the things you do in Colorado; snowmobiling, hunting, riding dirt bikes, and skiing. The risk of injury in the rugged mountains was therefore high. Dallenbach grabbed the bull by the horns shortly after moving there and began to develop an emergency medical system (EMS) for the small town of Basalt.

He convinced Bromley to return to school and become a paramedic to help expand the local program. Bromley excelled as a medic and soon reached supervisor status. Good EMS became a reality in Basalt as a result of these efforts. During this period, Dallenbach even purchased, and drove, a used ambulance all the way from New Jersey to Basalt so the town would have one.

Bromley was convinced to join the Safety Team as a paramedic in 1985. After becoming Director, he and Dallenbach worked diligently to enhance the image of the Team. No easy task. Local rescue personnel often looked at us as foreign invaders, unneeded, less than competent, and unwanted. Bromley began the very difficult task of regaining credibility and respect from the local track personnel. He eventually left Basalt for Wyoming, where he continued to teach other paramedics the art of advanced life support.

Being a medic in the remote areas of Wyoming and Colorado required stamina, innovation, and improvisation, all valuable skills on the race track. With Bromley in charge of safety, our reputation among the local medical providers improved considerably. We were no longer looked at as a 'necessary evil'. In fact, we were becoming very well respected and well tolerated. The team grew in size as well as in stature. We added two more trucks and 12 more men. Response time to crashes dropped to seconds even on the longer courses like the four-mile track at Elkhart Lake. Getting drivers out of their wrecked cars became a well defined skill. Specific tools, some actually designed by Bromley, enhanced this specialized form of rescue.

Bromley established drills at each event. We would go over difficult extrication scenarios and the proper use of the extrication tools and stabilization of the driver. We would invite the local medics to these sessions so that they could see and learn how specialized this form of rescue had become. The cars had grown more technically advanced through the years, with no wasted space. The driver had practically to be wedged into the car in order to drive. This made the extrication process more delicate and refined. Once very large, the older 'jaws' had been replaced with a newer model that was much smaller, lighter, and with more intricate attachments to clear a safe path to the entrapped driver.

By 1990, road courses shared equal billing with oval tracks in CART. The ovals, due to their much higher average speeds and the ever-present concrete wall, continued to be the most hazardous. Fewer crashes occurred on ovals than on road courses, but they were usually more severe. Road courses, in many respects, were more dangerous for the Safety Team members than for the drivers. That danger was inherent in the concept of what was called the 'local yellow'. On an oval, the track immediately goes 'full yellow' when a crash occurs. All the drivers slow down and maintain their positions. The pace car comes out and leads the field slowly and under control until the incident is cleared. On road courses the concept of the 'local yellow' applies. Road courses are usually longer than the oval tracks and with the many turns a paced field seems to take forever to complete a lap. Spectators despise full course yellows on road courses, much preferring the local yellow. During a local yellow, the drivers are supposed to slow down in the area of the crash. This simply does not happen. The area of the crash is defined for the drivers by flag-waving corner workers stationed before and after the incident.

We were forced by race control to work most road course crashes under a local yellow. Drivers unfortunately showed little regard for the waving yellow flags. The theory of the local yellow is good, but in reality, no one slows down! A driver is not voluntarily going to give up any ground he or she has gained during the course of a long and competitive race. In fact, workers in timing and scoring have often found that the fastest laps of the race have been run when there is a waving yellow flag somewhere on the course.

A local yellow in conjunction with a rainstorm is the worst possible scenario for the safety crew. Racecars do not crash in a predictable fashion when it rains. They will often appear to gain speed on wet grass due to a loss of friction provided by the pavement. In actuality they just don't slow down as fast. In addition, they frequently lose control in a direction opposite to what is usually anticipated. We have been fortunate in CART never to have injured or killed a Safety Team member as a result of contact with an errant racecar. But, in the Detroit, Michigan street race we came damn close!

Midway through the 1993 race, Michael Andretti, son of Mario, crashed into one of the tire barriers while leading. Bromley and I were immediately dispatched to the scene. We arrived at the wrecked car within seconds. Luckily, the younger Andretti was not hurt. His car could easily be towed out of harm's way so the incident was being treated as a local yellow by race control. The clean-up was completed rapidly and we handed Andretti the towrope for the ride back to the pits.

Meanwhile, Mario Andretti, also in contention for the lead, was speeding toward the crash site. In his calculating way, Mario had been trying to figure out on what lap we would be clear of the scene so he wouldn't have to lose any ground to the other drivers if he slowed down for Michael's crash.

He miscalculated! Just as we were beginning to pull away with Michael, Mario plowed into the rear of our truck at over 60 mph. I was tossed forward as a result of the impact, hitting my head on the rearview mirror. I couldn't believe what had happened. Some bozo had run into the Safety Truck! I jumped from the cab and ran to the back of the vehicle. There, I was shocked to find Mario wedged beneath our rear bumper. Another few inches and he could have been decapitated! Being focused and calculating are good traits for a race driver but this was ridiculous!

I was furious! The track was now blocked completely and a full-course yellow was called. I began to berate poor Mario. I called him every name in the book. Dutch driver Arie Luyendyk, forced to stop because of the crash, watched my behavior in amazement. He told me later he never thought a doctor could get that mad! My anger, I suspect, was more the result of fear because of how bad the incident could have been.

Mario was embarrassed. Michael wouldn't look at him. ESPN had a camera directly overhead and the whole sordid scene was caught on tape. The Safety Team busied themselves getting all the stalled cars back underway while I continued to gyrate aimlessly around the area.

As a result of the incident, the so-called 'Andretti' bumper was added to the rear of all of our Safety Trucks to prevent a recurrence. This new appendage was a flat, rectangular sheet of steel that extended down from the conventional bumper. Only three inches of ground clearance was allowed. In Mario's defense, he had simply miscalculated when to get back on the gas. A great race driver is continually plotting ways to gain a split-second advantage over the rest of the field. Sometimes he fails. Another two seconds and Mario would have made it, perhaps gaining a few precious seconds. He is still the driver of the century!

Chapter 21

A.J. Crashes at Elkhart Lake

S tepping back a bit in time, I want to mention another crash involving the legendary A.J. Foyt. It was August of 1991. We were racing in Elkhart Lake, Wisconsin on one of the most scenic and truly classic road courses anywhere. Over four miles in length, the track was the fastest road course in America and the longest. Several elevation changes, coupled with a large variety of corners, challenged drivers to the fullest. Many drivers describe Road America as their favorite track. Not A.J.

In the waning moments of his career, Foyt was running somewhere in the middle of the pack when his brakes apparently failed at the end of the long and very fast front straightaway. He was sent hurtling off the course at Turn One. He was going so fast that he cleared the gravel trap that had been put there to slow errant cars down, after becoming airborne. He did not slow down at all. He continued unabated and plowed into the dirt embankment that lined the end of the track's property line. The nosecone had been ripped from the car when he first left the track, turning the front of the car into a speeding backhoe. With his feet and legs exposed, the car burrowed into the mud all the way to Foyt's pelvis. Both legs were impacted by the dirt.

Dr. Trammell arrived on the scene in less than 30 seconds. He could hardly believe what he saw. The tip of one shoe was barely visible sticking out of the dirt impaction, the other shoe, and the rest of Foyt's legs, were nowhere to be seen. Foyt was wide awake and screaming in agony. Trammell began the first documented archeological dig in Indycar racing history. Not wanting to cause more damage than had already been done, he began painstakingly to spoon out small amounts of dirt a little bit at a time, searching for Foyt's missing limbs. The excavation took several minutes. In the meantime, Foyt was going crazy with pain.

Terry slowly began to uncover A.J.'s twisted and broken legs. Thankfully, all of the parts were still attached. Foyt continued to scream in agony. I was stationed in the medical center as usual and soon received a call from Terry on our private radio channel:

"Steve, can you come out here and bring some morphine?"

I jumped at the chance to go to the scene. I grabbed a vial of morphine and a syringe, leaped into our golf cart, and headed down the long front straight with Jon Potter at the helm. We were painfully slow, but finally arrived at the crash.

It was readily apparent that A.J. was in severe pain. His legs were badly fractured and Terry was still in the process of digging him out. I wrapped his arm with a tourniquet and gave him some morphine intravenously. This is practically unheard of in the field. First, surgeons don't like patients to have pain medicine before they're examined. This makes sense because pain medication might block a telltale neurological sign, masking an occult injury. Second, there is some risk to the patient's breathing mechanism when IV narcotics are given. And third, I was not licensed in the state of Wisconsin to administer medication outside of our medical unit. A.J. was very thankful in spite of the risks involved. He quieted down almost immediately and became much more cooperative. We carefully took him out of the car and placed him in the waiting helicopter. I had already summoned it to the scene before rushing out of the medical unit.

Terry and I were comfortable treating Foyt's pain in this way because we had all of the emergency equipment on hand to deal with a respiratory arrest should it occur. Also, we were sure that the injuries to his legs were his only ones. Stating again that he was "too old for this shit", Foyt recovered at Methodist Hospital and went on to race for a couple more years. He retired on Pole Day at Indianapolis in 1993.

Chapter 22

THE BLACK BOXES

In 1992 Dr. Trammell and I were approached by the Motorsports Research Group at General Motors. Tommy Kendall, an up-and-coming young Californian driver, had been involved in a huge crash during the International Motor Sports Association (IMSA) race at Watkins Glen, New York earlier in the year. The car he was driving was a high-performance, very sophisticated, prototype sportscar. It had little in the way of front-end protection. He had badly fractured both legs as a result of the crash. At the request of Kendall's family, General Motors had been asked to investigate the cause of the accident thoroughly. The division at GM that was put in charge of this was under the control of a man named John Pierce. Pierce was one of the first from the automobile industry to acknowledge the fact that there was something to be learned from open-wheeled racecars that routinely crash at over 200 mph and, more often than not, allow the driver to emerge unscathed.

Pierce's department normally concerned itself with the study of highway crashes only. Using high-tech biomechanical models, his department reconstructed crashes in order to improve the design of passenger cars and trucks. The department's crash and injury reconstruction studies were led by Dr. John Melvin, a world authority on crash/injury cause and effect. Both Pierce and Melvin felt that highway safety could benefit from the scientific investigation of racecar crashes.

Pierce arranged a meeting at Sir Winston's restaurant on board the *Queen Mary* during the Long Beach Grand Prix in 1992. Dr. Trammell, John Melvin, Kirk Russell, CART's technical director, and I were invited to attend. Following a lengthy discussion on the merits of using the CART series as a laboratory of sorts, the group from GM offered to supply and maintain crash recorders for our cars. Trammell and I were ecstatic. Similar to the black boxes in airplanes, these recorders would collect impact data in real time that could be downloaded later for crash reconstruction. They housed a tri-axial accelerometer arrangement that would allow us to measure the magnitude of the forces involved in a crash in three directions, vertical, horizontal, and longitudinal. This information would allow the development of highly sophisticated computer models enabling us to re-enact our injury-producing crashes in the laboratory. We could then alter variables in car construction and equipment design that would, in turn, lead to improved protection in the cars without endangering a driver's life. For the first time, we would now be able to marry injury-producing trends with what actually happens to the cars, and make design changes based on scientific fact and not someone's gut feeling. The CART Board gave the project their unanimous approval and later that year recorders were placed in a few of our cars for trial. We immediately began to collect truly meaningful crash and impact data.

One of the injury trends that Trammell and I had recently noticed was an alarming increase in the number of pelvic and hip injuries over the preceding three years. We were seeing these injuries after especially big crashes on the ovals. Racecars were impacting the walls sideways with greater frequency, subjecting the driver's vulnerable hip and pelvic areas to severe compressive forces. This shift in impact angle from the standard frontal crash allowed the gearshift lever, located next to the driver's right hip, to embed itself into the driver's thigh. Several broken femurs and fractured pelvises had occurred as a result.

Rick Mears offered the most plausible explanation for this change in impact angle. He reasoned that instead of spinning 360 degrees prior to impact as before, the cars were now rotating less than 270 degrees. This change in rotation was due to faster cornering speeds. There was simply not enough time to spin all the way around before crashing. He attributed this shorter spin arc to improved adhesion from better tires and the greater downforce developed by the engineers. Engineering data confirmed that the corner speeds had indeed increased over the years.

Rules makers, in their never-ending attempt to slow the cars down, usually succeeded in controlling straightaway speeds only. Speed in a straightline was much the same in 1993 as it was in 1960. The old Novi racecars were reportedly clocked at over 230 mph on the backstretch at Indianapolis during the early 60s. After reviewing the accumulated crash data, our technical committee announced a number of rule changes designed to increase the integrity of the tub against side impact. They also announced alterations to the location of the gearshift lever inside the car. The incidence of hip and pelvic injury was soon reduced as a result.

Data continued to pour in from the crash boxes. We learned that a human being, properly restrained, could survive an impact of more than 100 G. Previously published data from sled tests in the 50s claimed that 50 G was the upper limit of human tolerance. We were learning more from our crash recorders than we could assimilate easily. Properly interpreting the data required specialized knowledge. We soon developed a close working relationship with a number of accomplished biomechanical engineers including not only Dr. Melvin, but also Dr. Ted Knox, Dr. Pria Prasad, and Dr. Robert Hubbard. Knox was head of biomechanical research at Wright-Patterson Air Force Base in Dayton, Ohio. Prasad was head of biomechanical research at Ford Motor Co., and Hubbard was a professor of biomechanics at Michigan State. Hubbard was the designer of the most often used crash test dummy head, and Melvin was instrumental in the first use of air bags.

As more data was analyzed, more changes were made to the cars. Suspension geometry was changed to decrease the chance of intrusion of parts into the cockpit. Alterations were also made to the sidepods. Changes were based now on fact and not fancy. With the crash recorders installed in all of the cars in 1993, motorsports safety had entered a new era.

Chapter 23

THE COMING OF NIGEL

Drivers in the early to mid-90s were entering the CART series from all parts of the world. Formula One, the world's premier racing series, had a very limited number of seats and CART was the next most desirable series for future stars. As a consequence young, talented drivers with F1 aspirations like Jacques Villeneuve clamored to enter CART. In addition older, accomplished champions like Fittipaldi were also coming in. The attraction for the older drivers was an extension of their career and a chance actually to have some fun racing. Formula One was well known for its intensity and very stressful environment. The European drivers frequently complained that it was "not much fun anymore". One of these new, older drivers to enter CART was Nigel Mansell. He was the reigning World Champion! He had just come off a spectacular season in Formula One and much to everyone's surprise had agreed to leave to drive in CART. In 1993 he would drive for the powerful Newman-Haas Racing team owned by movie star Paul Newman and entrepreneur Carl Haas.

Recently appointed as a special constable on the Isle of Man, Mansell had risen to the pinnacle of racing success in a very few years. Revered by fans all over Europe, he was one of the most popular of all Formula One champions. He, like Fittipaldi, took the CART series by storm, and immediately started to win races. He was the first CART driver to ever win a coveted pole position in his rookie year. Ovals or road courses, it didn't seem to matter. Nigel was exceptionally fast!

His team-mate in the Newman-Haas stable was racing legend Mario Andretti. Mansell and Andretti did not seem to be the best of friends. For unknown reasons, a fierce rivalry soon developed between the two of them. Perhaps it was simply the fact that they had each won the Formula One World Championship and there was a lingering question as to who might be the better driver. A rivalry among competitive team-mates was a huge delight for the fans, but could be a royal pain in the ass for the team and its owners.

Mansell won his first-ever oval race on the high banks of the treacherous Michigan Speedway, beating Mario who came in a distant second. No one could remember anyone else ever able to do this. The weather that day was excruciatingly hot, with many of the drivers complaining. Mansell not only complained about the heat, but also complained constantly over his radio during the race about having a headache and not feeling well.

When, after driving brilliantly, he pulled into Victory Lane, he needed help getting out of the car. Andretti, who had just driven the same number of miles, in the same searing heat, spryly popped out of his car. Mansell had radioed his crew shortly before the end of the race asking for iced towels and medical assistance to greet him at the finish.

After rolling slowly to a stop near the podium, he staggered limply from his car. His fans gasped! He appeared to be having some difficulty getting his breath. Meanwhile, Andretti was vibrantly entertaining his crew as well as members of the media, seemingly unaffected by the rigors of the race. Dr. Trammell and I had also been alerted to Nigel's complaint of exhaustion. Worried, we both rushed to the podium as soon as the checkered flag fell. When we arrived, we found him slumped forlornly against the victory backdrop, his head wrapped in cold towels. Andretti was staring at him, appearing somewhat confused. Mansell slumped further into the backdrop and some in attendance swear they caught a glimpse of a wink. Suddenly, as if struck from some divine influence, he began to recover from his apoplectic state. With renewed vigor, he rose slowly to his feet and began waving to the delighted crowd. He grabbed a British flag and hoisted it high above his head with both arms and waved it back and forth triumphantly.

Nigel, I think, is so competitive that he uses every device he can muster to win races and market his skills, including the psychological. There is an advantage to be had if one can convince their opponent of some frailty. Appearing to be exhausted left no doubt in the minds of the fans that he had given his all for Queen and Country. Call him a master showman or whatever you like, he is an unbelievably talented racing driver, the likes of which have only been seen on rare occasions.

Earlier that year, Nigel had been involved in a major crash at Phoenix. It was his first on an oval track. He lost control of his car during practice at over 170 mph while exiting the first turn. According to one of his crew members, his approach to high-speed driving in the past had always been to push his car to its limit, and then slightly beyond so he new exactly how fast he could take a certain corner. This approach worked reasonably well on wide-open road courses with a lot of run-off area, but not so well when an unforgiving concrete wall loomed close at hand.

He hit the outer wall of Turn 1 hard, so hard that the gearbox actually penetrated the six inches of concrete. After impact, a gaping hole in the wall several inches wide revealed the crystal blue Arizona sky. It was a massive rear impact. As the wall grabbed his gearbox, a tremendous shearing force tore at his lower back. The force of the crash rendered him senseless. The damage to the car was severe and made for a difficult extrication.

As we were getting him out of the car, I radioed for the helicopter. We took Nigel straight from the scene of the crash to the heliport. I jumped into the helicopter along with Rosanne, his charming and classically beautiful wife. Riding in a helicopter was still not my favorite thing to do. Mansell woke up soon after we arrived in the emergency room. He didn't know me from the man in the moon. At first, he didn't recognize Rosanne either. He soon became agitated, not uncommon following a concussion, and loudly insisted that he be released. It took several minutes for Rosanne and me to calm him down. Overnight observation in the hospital for any driver known to have been unconscious was mandatory. I had put that policy into effect after hearing of an incident years earlier involving Formula One and Indycar/Can Am champion driver Mark Donohue.

Donohue was driving for Roger Penske's team in 1975 and had a big crash during the pre-race morning warm-up session for the Austrian Grand Prix at the Osterreichring. He sustained a heavy blow to the head from a scaffold pole from an advertising banner, but after getting out of his car was able to hold a lucid conversation with Emerson Fittipaldi, among others, before being helicoptered to the hospital. He died a few days later, just as everybody was feeling grateful that he had survived. The autopsy revealed a large blood clot on his brain that had slowly enlarged to the point of killing him.

After explaining this to a much calmer Mansell, he reluctantly agreed to remain in the hospital overnight. He was released early the next morning. Sore, but undaunted, he returned by private jet to his Florida residence. Once home, he soon developed a rather intimate relationship with Dr. Trammell and me. This was the result of the treatment he required for an injury we had never seen before.

A large collection of fluid had developed rapidly beneath the skin of his lower lumbar region shortly after the crash. It continued to grow in size after he returned home. It grew so large, in fact, that it affected his daily activities, especially his ability to play golf, his favorite thing to do when he wasn't racing. The accumulated fluid in his back was the result of the tremendous shearing forces he had experienced during the crash. The soft tissues of his lumbar area were torn and shredded beneath his skin under the severe strain. This separation of the tissues allowed fluid to accumulate among the many layers.

Dr. Trammell would later name this the 'Mansell Lesion'. The only description of a similar one we could find was from a pathologist who described it in deceased victims of plane crashes. So much fluid would seep into Nigel's lower back that he required needle drainage on an almost daily basis. When at a race, either

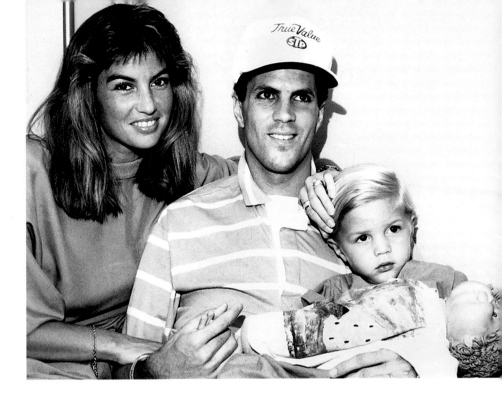

Roberto Guerrero with wife Kati and son Marco, upon his release from Methodist Hospital in 1987. (Author)

Roberto Guerrero with the author at Phoenix in 1988, both pondering whether he should be there. (Dan R. Boyd)

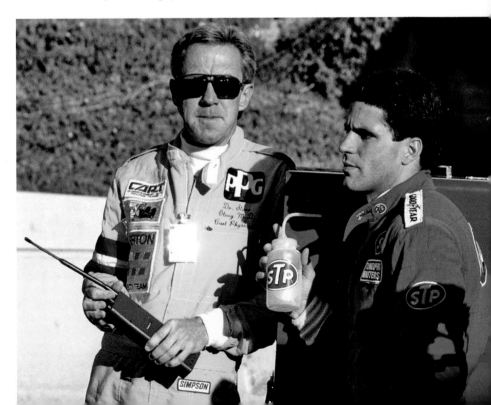

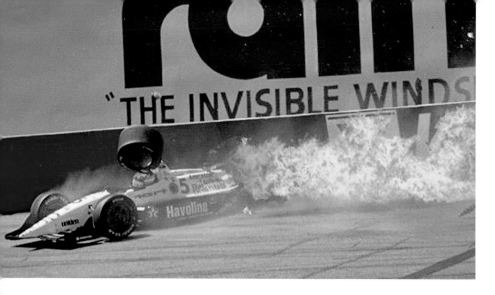

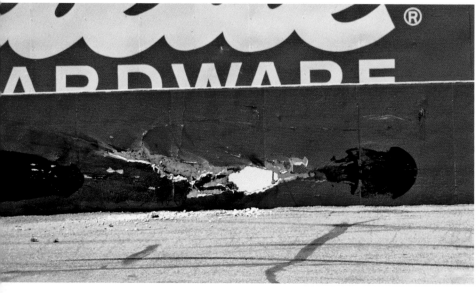

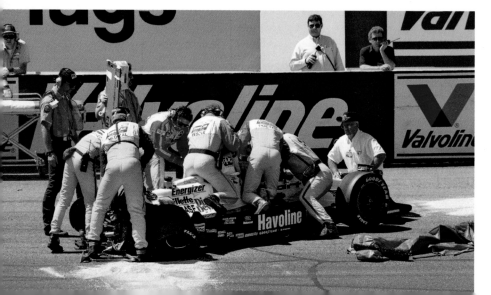

OPPOSITE TOP *Nigel Mansell pounds the wall during testing at Phoenix in 1993.* (LesWelch.com)

OPPOSITE MIDDLE *The hole punched through six inches of concrete by Mansell's gearbox reveals the clear Arizona sky.* (LesWelch.com)

OPPOSITE BOTTOM *Mansell's extrication from the wreckage at Phoenix.* (LesWelch.com)

RIGHT *Original medic Jerry Guise and the venerable MR-10.* (Dan R. Boyd)

BELOW *Emerson Fittipaldi was nearly paralyzed by this 1996 accident at Michigan.* (Author)

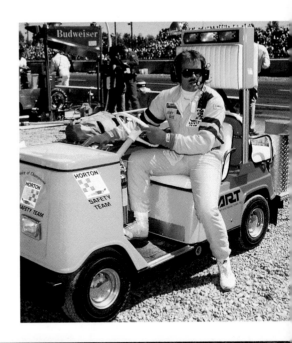

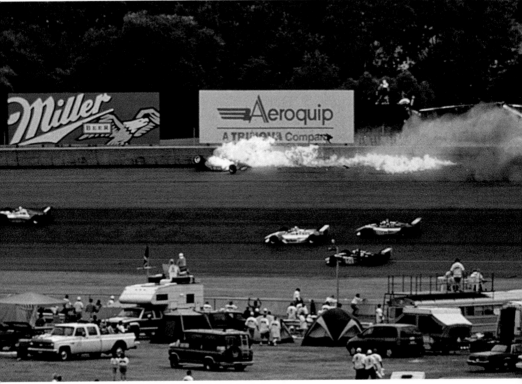

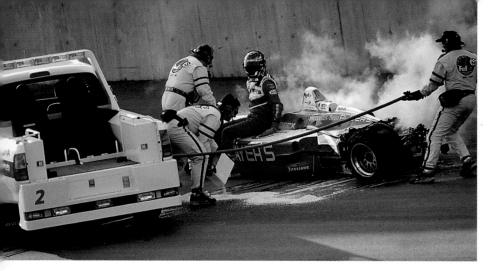

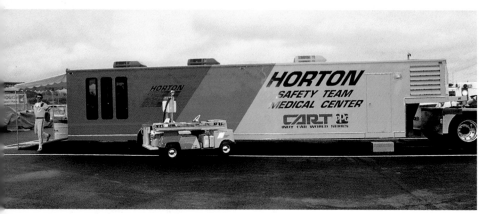

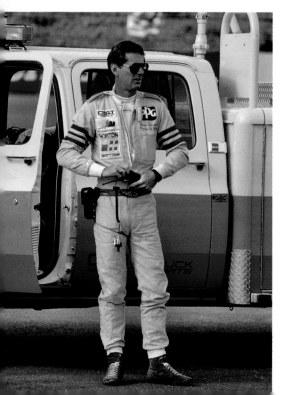

Top *Greg Moore demonstrates the calm demeanor of the professional driver following a big crash.* (Dan R. Boyd)

Middle *Our first purpose-built medical unit in 1986, compliments of Carl Horton.* (Dan R. Boyd)

Left *Steve Edwards, CART's first Safety Director.* (Dan R. Boyd)

Opposite top *Our second purpose-built medical unit in 1989.* (Dan R. Boyd)

Opposite bottom *Members of the CART Safety Team salute the drivers as they begin the 1994 Road America race at Elkhart Lake, Wisconsin.* (Dan R. Boyd)

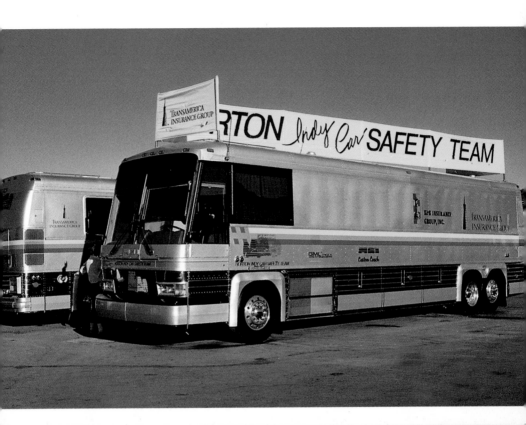

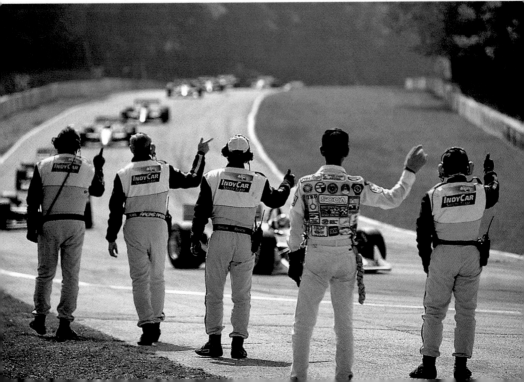

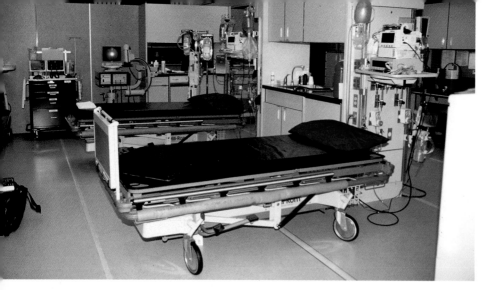

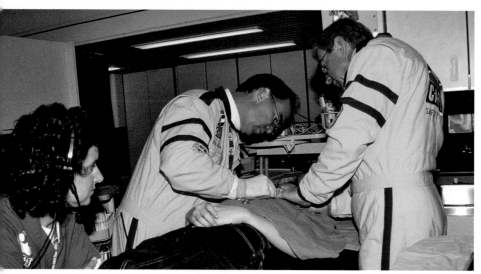

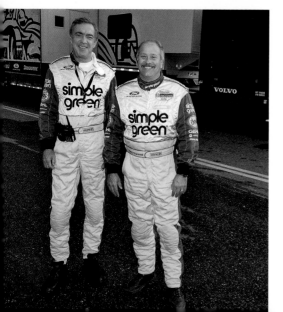

Top *Inside the third and final CART medical unit in 1996 – the ultimate!* (Dan R. Boyd)

Middle *Dr. Rick Timms and the author perform minor surgery inside the new medical unit.* (Dan R. Boyd)

Left *The author and Dr. Terry Trammell, happy the day is over.* (Dan R. Boyd)

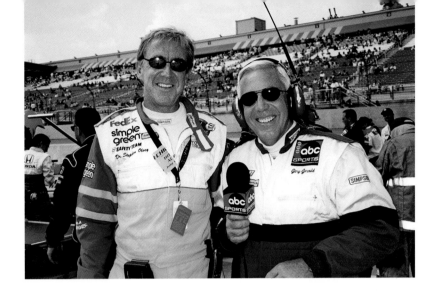

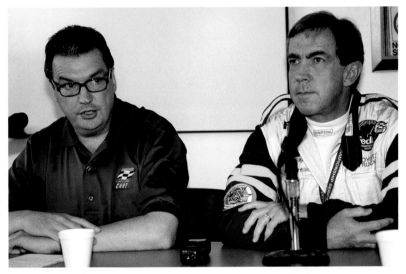

Top *The author with favorite announcer, Gary Gerould.* (Author)

Middle *Explaining the death of young driver Gonzalo Rodriguez at Laguna Seca in 1999 as CART's CEO, Andrew Craig, looks on.* (Motorsport Images)

Right *Greg Moore with his fractured finger in ice, the day before he died at the California Speedway, in 1999.* (Author)

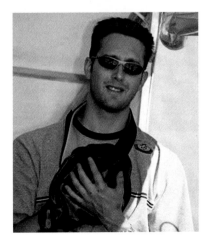

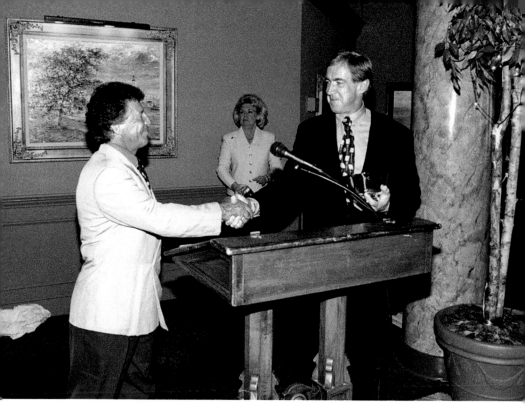

ABOVE *The author receives the Mario Andretti Award from the man himself; the Driver of the Century.* (Author)

BELOW *Hanging out with the cast of the movie* Driven *following the day's shoot. Actors Sylvester Stallone, Cristián de la Fuente and Kip Pardue are pictured.* (Author)

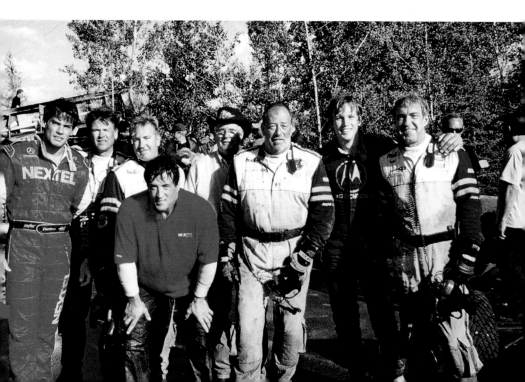

Terry or I would stick a large needle into him and drain up to one liter of fluid at a time. We continued this treatment for several weeks as he was determined to remain competitive and not miss any races.

We would drain him in the office, in hotel rooms, in our medical unit, and in his motorhome. He continued to race in spite of the marked pain and discomfort he experienced following the Phoenix crash and qualified well for the Indy 500 that May. Nigel Mansell was as tough as they come. On raceday, we planned to drain his back just prior to the start of the 500 so that he would begin the long and arduous event with as little fluid in his back as possible.

I wasn't particularly busy raceday morning, and was in the process of draining Mansell's back inside his motorhome when my wife suddenly burst through the front door. She had not yet had the pleasure of meeting Nigel. Earlier that morning, he had told me to have Lynne stop by so that they could be formally introduced. Her timing could not have been better. An unobstructed view of Nigel's behind greeted her as she boisterously popped through the front door. Without changing his position or the expression on his face, and showing little in the way of surprise, he slowly reached around, extended his hand, and said in a very matter-of-fact way:

"Hello there, I'm Nigel, very pleased to meet you."

For the first time I could remember, Lynne was speechless. I completed the procedure while she and Nigel carried on an animated conversation about life in Indy during the month of May. Nigel soon left to prepare for the start of the race. Lynne's color didn't return to normal until much later in the day.

By 1994, Terry's and my relationship with the Speedway had become somewhat strained. We were referred to by friends as "the bastards at the family picnic". We were supposed to be there, but no one in 'the family' really wanted us. The old guard in USAC was bitter over the fact that the CART drivers were dominating their prize event. In their minds our newer, non-American drivers failed to show the proper respect due the

Speedway. Fittipaldi upset them greatly when he drank orange juice instead of the traditional bottle of milk after winning the race in 1989. The CART teams and drivers would show up each year in early May, practice, qualify, race, and then take the majority of the Speedway's money and go on down the road to Milwaukee. Trammell and I were the only CART officials to have any sort of position at all at the Speedway.

Animosity also grew on the Speedway's Safety Team. I was asked by Dr. Bock to quit working on the race track in 1990. Trammell and I were both discouraged from practicing within the track's hospital. The bitterness grew so severe that when one of our patients went to the care center looking for us, the receptionist denied that we were on the Speedway's medical staff. During the race itself, we were relegated to a narrow grassy strip located just inside of Turns 1 and 2. There, we would anxiously wait to go to Methodist Hospital if one of our drivers became injured. We had the proper credentials, but were expected to keep a very low profile while inside the Speedway's confines.

We were keeping this low profile when Mansell was nearly beheaded by driver Dennis Vittolo. Vittolo, a great guy but not a great race driver, had somehow managed to drive his car up and over the top of Mansell's car on the pit access road while Mansell was coming in for a routine pit stop. Nigel appeared to be unhurt in the incident, but was taken by ambulance to the infield hospital for the mandatory examination.

When he arrived inside the care center, the nursing staff told him to lie down on one of the beds. They then swarmed over him to begin their compulsory examination. Mansell knew he wasn't hurt and was very angry at having been knocked so needlessly out of the race, so he resisted their attention. The nurses were relentless but Mansell would have none of it. He reportedly got off of the bed and ran to the other side of the examining room, upsetting a tray of supplies as he reached the far wall. He backed up against the wall to face the befuddled nursing staff. He then began yelling for me as he fended off the approaching horde of medical workers.

This may be a slight exaggeration of the facts, but I did receive a frantic call from Hank's excellent assistant, Mary Simpson, to go to the infield hospital as soon as possible.

When I arrived there, Nigel stood with his back against the wall yelling at the nurses to leave him alone. It was all I could do not to laugh. Professional drivers, in my experience, usually know when they're hurt and when they're not, as long as they have their wits about them. Nigel was completely lucid. In their defense, many of the nurses at the Speedway had never worked any races outside of Indianapolis. As a consequence, they were a bit over-zealous in rendering care to drivers who were uninjured. Most of the drivers politely put up with the added attention out of respect for the event and the overall excellent care that they receive in a true emergency. The highly competitive Mansell was extremely angry that he was out of a race that he was likely going to win, and was in no mood to placate the young nursing staff. He was the odds-on favorite and his forced retirement from competition was an atrocity.

I attempted to calm him down. After a few minutes, he hesitantly agreed to a cursory examination. I negotiated a deal with the staff not to stick him with any needles and to allow him to disrobe in peace. After the exam, we left the compound with Nigel grumbling obscenities at the two yellow-shirted gate guards who were unnecessarily blowing their whistles at us as we crossed the road.

Mansell had won the CART Championship the previous year, winning five races and seven pole positions. His total share of the prize money that year was over 2.5 million dollars. He was without question the best out-of-the-box driver ever to hit the CART series. His subtle, quick-witted humor was a constant treat for those around him. When you were with Nigel, you knew who was in charge. Unlike so many drivers of the modern era, he was very appreciative of the efforts put forth on his behalf, and he let you know it. He left the CART series after '94, returning briefly to the highly charged environment of Formula One. He remains a good friend, and I truly believe he will continue competing at something until he can no longer get out of bed.

The Mansell incident didn't help my situation in USAC. The hostility toward CART in general continued to build. Open-wheeled racing, and CART in particular, was enjoying its highest level of popularity. Stands were full at most, if not all of the events, and TV ratings were steadily climbing. Internally, it was a very different story. Politics and greed were beginning to fragment the sport and had reached its peak by 1995. Sadly, that would be the last great year at the Indianapolis Motor Speedway.

Lined up for the start of the '95 race were Michael Andretti, son of Mario, and Christian Fittipaldi, nephew of Emerson. Jacques Villeneuve, Gil de Ferran, Arie Luyendyk and Bobby Rahal were there, as were former Formula One drivers Mauricio Gugelmin, Danny Sullivan, Eddie Cheever, Roberto Guerrero, Teo Fabi, Stefan Johansson and Eliseo Salazar. Missing from the line-up were former Formula One World Champion Emerson Fittipaldi and Al Unser Jr. The powerful Penske team surprisingly failed to qualify for Indy, the biggest race in the world. There was record attendance and TV ratings were at their peak. Villeneuve beat the stellar field, winning the famous race at his second attempt.

Shortly after that race Tony George, the president of the Indianapolis Motor Speedway, dropped the big bomb. He announced that he was going to split open-wheel racing! George decreed that the Indianapolis 500 Mile Race would no longer be open to the CART teams; the teams that had dominated the event since 1979. He announced a new entity that he called the Indy Racing League, IRL. The 'League' was to become a George-owned sanctioning body for an all-American series, to be run exclusively on oval tracks. It was designed to be much more affordable than the outrageously expensive CART series. According to George, it would not be influenced by either the automakers or the engine companies. It was to be a haven for young American sprint and midget car drivers wishing to break into the big time. In other words, it was an attempt to turn back the sands of time.

George, I think, had been had by the likes of A.J. Foyt, Rick Galles, and Dick Simon, whose teams were no longer competitive in CART. They all wanted things to be like they were in the 60s. John Menard, a wealthy hardware store owner from Wisconsin, was involved as well. Menard raced his cars only at Indy. Other former car owners and participants from the CART series had also become disgruntled with CART's arrogant elite and helped to convince George he was doing the right thing.

The general feeling in Indianapolis, according to the *Indianapolis Star*, was that the highly successful superteam owned by Roger Penske had driven everyone else in CART out of competition, therefore making the IRL more desirable. Many wondered if NASCAR might have influenced George to some degree. NASCAR would definitely stand to benefit if open-wheel was torn apart. At the time of the announcement, CART was actually outdrawing NASCAR at their shared events. The George decision was arguably one of the worst things to happen to open-wheeled racing in the history of the sport.

Splitting Indycar racing into two series ultimately split the fan base. Many fans became hopelessly disgruntled and changed their allegiance to NASCAR. Many more left automobile racing altogether. NASCAR began to expand exponentially while open-wheeled racing shriveled. Life in both series would soon change drastically.

Chapter 24

ANOTHER NEW
MEDICAL UNIT

In the fall of 1995, while Tony George was putting the final plans in place for his new series, Terry and I decided we needed another new medical unit. Patient visits had continued to increase and we needed more versatility and room. We planned our new unit in the quaint, dimly lit bar at the Hotel La Playa in Carmel, California after our season-ending race at Laguna Seca. We were now routinely treating more than 70 patients a weekend. Also, the current unit was in need of some expensive major repairs. We were cramped and needed space to expand our program. We wanted the ability to care for up to six ill or injured patients at a time.

In addition to our acute care capabilities, we also offered physical therapy to injured drivers and other participants through an organization of athletic trainers sponsored by the Justin Boot Company. The therapists were under the direction of trainer Don Andrews and were operating out of a truck parked in proximity, but not always next to, our medical unit. Andrews had been providing therapy to professional rodeo cowboys for years. He had a team of well-respected and very experienced trainers working for him. We wanted Andrews' bunch to become an integral part of our medical system and needed a unit large enough to include them.

After a couple of vodkas, Trammell and I grabbed some cocktail napkins and began to design a new unit, formulating our wishlist. We included all the equipment and supplies we would need to take care of any imaginable crash scenario. We added a proper communications and reception area and our own bathroom. We planned adequate space for the trainers and room for the nurses to function more freely. It soon became apparent that a fullsize semi-trailer truck with expandable sides would be required to satisfy all of our wants. We were aware of mobile MRI scanners and cardiac catheterization units already on the road so we felt an emergency care center could be made to fit such a platform. With fingers crossed we submitted our plans to the CART Board of Directors.

I thought we would be lucky to get half of what we wanted from them. Surprisingly, we received a favorable response. The problem now became who could build such a unit? No such facility existed anywhere in the world. Wally Dallenbach as Chief Steward was very supportive of our request and just happened to know a couple of guys from Colorado who had been in the hospital-building business. The Board authorized the formation of a company whose sole responsibility was to build our new unit. Appropriately enough, it was named the Colorado Medical Company.

A design process ensued with Terry, the builders, and me passing renderings back and forth for six months. The technicalities of designing a mobile care center of this magnitude were substantial. For example, Terry and I wanted hanging lights like they have in hospitals to illuminate the exam and surgical areas. The builders pointed out that such lights would be severed at their origin when the unit was hydraulically closed for travel. Whoops!

Everything in the unit, cabinets and all, needed to fit together like a puzzle in order for the unit to close properly. Otherwise it would become one of the world's most expensive trash mashers. Terry made a number of trips to the building site while I went on a search for the necessary equipment.

As luck would have it, two years earlier I had met a very dynamic sales woman named Kimbra O'Krinski. She had burst into my office one day in Miami in an attempt to sell me a new blood gas analyzer for our intensive care unit. O'Krinski, it turned out, was connected in some fashion to almost every medical device manufacturer in the United States as well as most of those abroad. Formerly with NASA as a flight nurse, she had clawed her way up the corporate sales ladder to a prominent position in one of the latest spin-off high-tech medical companies.

I called and asked if she would help us obtain some cardiac monitors, a ventilator, blood pressure machines, a rapid blood infuser, and all the other necessary high-tech equipment. She said sure, and what's more she stated that she would also obtain all of the expendable materials, such as bandages, needles and sutures we would need. Three months later, O'Krinski had promoted over $185,000 worth of supplies and state-of-the-art equipment. The CART medical unit was going to have better monitoring equipment than most hospitals in the country. Not only did Ms. O'Krinski acquire the equipment, she also managed to have it donated with no strings attached for a period of five years with a full warranty and replacement contract for each item! We were in business!

The new unit was put into service in 1996. We now had over 850 square feet of air-conditioned space with more than enough headroom. We could accommodate four super-sick patients at a time with room in the rear for the trainers. If needed, we could convert the rear section into two more acute care beds. We had a permanent, two-bed critical care area, a reception area, and the nurses had their own workstation. It was the only mobile unit like it in the world. The total value was well over one million dollars!

Included in the equipment was a small fluoroscopy unit that allowed us to X-ray 90% of the orthopedic injuries that occurred on any given race weekend. This ability saved CART and the race teams a considerable amount of money. Instead of having to send an injured crewman along with someone to drive him back from the hospital for X-rays at a prohibitive cost, we could simply rule out or diagnose a fracture in our mobile unit, for free. Very often we could return the injured crewman to competition within minutes. With all of the emergency equipment on board, we felt that we could confidently handle any immediate life-threatening situation.

You name it we saw it. Even team owner/actor Paul Newman

had to visit our new medical center. He had accidentally cut off the end of his left middle finger while preparing a salad in his hospitality tent for some invited guests. He calmly left his guests and rode his motor scooter through the crowded paddock to the medical center, bleeding as he went.

Our nurses cleaned and dressed the wound as he woefully explained that he sure hoped the end of his finger hadn't made anyone ill. After a brief conversation about past racing experiences, he left the unit with his left hand proudly elevated as instructed and his middle finger prominently extended for all to see. As he walked out the door he cheerfully remarked:

"I've been wanting to show this finger to a lot of people, for a long, long time."

Chapter 25

CART GOES IT ALONE
AND TRAGEDY STRIKES

The Indy Racing League began operations over the winter of 1995. CART and the IRL entered the 1996 season as totally separate entities. For CART, it was largely business as usual with only two of its regular teams having defected. Dick Simon and A.J. Foyt went to the other side. As May approached, the CART Board of Directors bravely decided to run an independent race on the same day as, and in competition with, the Indianapolis 500. They planned the new event for the dangerous and infamous Michigan International Speedway. They would call the event the 'US 500'.

Many racing notables thought this decision was suicidal. Remarkably, 110,000 people were on hand for the start of the inaugural event. The race was run under tremendous scrutiny by the media with the obvious comparison being made to the IRL. CART felt that they had the best drivers in the world and they publicized that fact in their pre-race advertising. The morning of the race the drivers were really wired. The eyes of the entire racing world were focused on the event. The day dawned windy, damp, and miserably cold. "We're going to show those people on 16th street!" was the commonly heard war cry.

The race started amid the usual pre-race hoopla. On the very first lap prominent Mexican driver, Adrian Fernandez, the pole position driver, lost control of his car midway between the third and fourth turns. A huge nine-car pile-up ensued. The crash unfolded as if in slow motion. No one seemed able to get out of anyone else's way. To the unknowing, the drivers looked like complete idiots.

Thankfully, no one was hurt physically in the carnage that followed. Of the nine drivers involved, seven were able to get back in the race, most using back-up cars. The irreversible damage, however, had been done! CART's collective pride suddenly hit rock bottom. The clean-up process seemed to take forever due to the massive amount of debris scattered over the track. CART's embarrassment was broadcast live on national TV and vehemently ridiculed in the national press. The sad incident prophetically set the tone for the rest of the year.

In June, Trammell and I found ourselves in busy and fun downtown Toronto for the annual race held along the waterfront. The stands were full and it was a beautiful sunny day; a perfect day for a race. I was sitting as usual next to Lon Bromley in Safety 1 at the end of the long gently curving backstretch. Terry was in Safety 2 located upstream at the beginning of the same straight. The race until then had been largely uneventful, with Adrian Fernandez looking like a sure winner with only three laps to go. I was tired and ready to go back to the hotel; in a hurry to get out of my steaming firesuit. Like many of the street races, the event had been fairly boring. Very little passing had occurred. It was more a parade than a race. I was thinking ahead to the drivers' party planned for later that evening.

Due to where I was seated in the truck and to our location on the track, I could not see the cars coming toward us very well. My view was blocked by the concrete barrier and the catchfencing angled in front of the truck to protect us from any flying bits of debris. I was suddenly shocked to attention by a high-speed blur to my left. What looked like a bunch of errant car parts had pelted the adjacent tire barrier. I immediately jumped from the truck and ran toward the barrier. It initially appeared that three cars were locked together in the tires. Emerson Fittipaldi's car was one of them. I rushed to the crash site. As I approached, it became apparent that there were actually only two complete cars. What I thought was a third car was just an engine and gearbox assembly lying twisted and smoldering among the wreckage.

Confirming that Fittipaldi and the other driver were uninjured, I looked back up the track to check for oncoming traffic and to see where the rest of the third car might be. To my horror, I realized that a badly wrecked tub lay crumpled against the outside retaining wall several yards away. Bromley had seen the original collision at the head of the straightaway, very near the location of Safety 2. What he observed was one car being launched into the air off another one. The launched car nearly cleared the debris fence and appeared to have pushed the fence into a nearby tree. Contained by the fence, the car bounced back on to the pavement in two distinct pieces.

The car, we found out later, had been broken in two by the large tree. Both halves, one containing the engine and gearbox, the other containing the driver, then slid rapidly after impact toward the location of Safety 1. The half with the driver in it stopped about 40 yards up course. The engine and gearbox continued into the tire barrier to our left. My colleagues, seeing the crash happen, had rushed immediately to the remains of the car upstream.

With a sickening feeling, I ran toward the crumpled tub. The others were frantically engaged in a massive rescue effort. The driver of the car was still strapped in his seat. As I approached the crash site, it became apparent that Jeff Krosnoff, the young, fast Californian driving for Cal Wells, wasn't moving. By the time I arrived, his helmet had been removed and one of the Safety Team members was working feverishly to secure his airway. He was not breathing. Oxygen had been started. With his helmet off, I could see that he had sustained massive injuries to his head. Later investigation and review of the video showed that Krosnoff's head had likely made direct contact with the tree that had torn the car in half.

His pupils did not react and he was not responding to any kind of stimulation. He was chalky white in color. He was dead. Trammell arrived in Safety 2. By then, I had called in a 'Code 10'. This is the code number we assign to a fatality. We have only four codes to describe the initial condition of a driver, 1, 3, 5, and 10.

1 is no injury at all, 3 is a possible injury, 5 is a potentially life-threatening injury, and 10 is a fatality. This was the first time I had ever called in a code 10.

Terry and I needed to establish a patent airway in order to continue the pretext that we were trying to resuscitate the driver. We could no longer simply breathe for him with a bag and mask because his airway was totally obstructed with blood and other debris. We were certainly not going to declare him at the scene and encounter the fiasco we had with Gordon Smiley years ago at the Speedway. No one dies at the race track unless he or she is decapitated or incinerated.

We yelled for our airway kit. One of our medics grabbed it from the truck and ran toward us. As he approached, he slipped on the oily surface and fell to the pavement. The kit slid out of anyone's reach. Thinking fast, Terry grabbed a Leatherman multiple use tool from medic Mike Carey. Simultaneously, I grabbed a pair of hemostats out of the pocket in the front of my uniform. We began an emergency tracheotomy.

Terry made a horizontal slit in Jeff's throat. I then separated the exposed tissues with the hemostat while Terry quickly located the trachea (windpipe). A hole was punched in the trachea and we shoved the tube into place. We attached the oxygen and began to breathe for him. An ESPN camera crew caught the entire procedure on film. They later told us that we took only 19 seconds to secure the airway.

We then gingerly extricated Krosnoff and placed him in the waiting ambulance. I jumped in while continuing to squeeze the bag rhythmically, expecting to head directly for the hospital where he could be declared officially dead. It had been a long time since anything this tragic had happened.

Medical management for the Toronto race is under the very capable direction of Dr. Hugh Scully. Dr. Scully is a prominent cardiovascular surgeon in Toronto and a pre-eminent physician in Canada. He is a Professor of Surgery at the University of Toronto and Medical Director for Molson's sports marketing organization, the main sponsor of the event. He has been instrumental in organizing and providing medical care at Canadian race tracks for years. From a medical standpoint, the Toronto event was exceptionally well managed except for one lingering thorn in Scully's side. He had been plagued with a peculiar political problem in the province of Ontario for years. The Ontario Race Physicians, an organization formed to provide medical care at Ontario race tracks, had managed to acquire the exclusive rights to the provision of on-track ambulance service instead of using the municipal ambulance service. Only their specially equipped vehicles, not city ambulances, could be used for on-track rescue. This system likely developed because of reluctance on the part of city ambulance attendants to expose themselves to the dangers of on-track rescue years before.

Dr. Scully had been forced to live with this rule since its inception. As a result, I had to place Krosnoff's body in an ambulance that was not legally allowed to travel on public roads. Consequently, the driver made a meaningless lap of the entire race circuit because, I think, he was embarrassed to tell me that he could not drive on city streets.

This needless lap allowed just enough time for Krosnoff's family to organize themselves in a private car, and to fall in behind the city ambulance that eventually arrived to take us off the grounds. I was so angry by the time we finally got into the second ambulance that I lost my voice from yelling at the driver. I consequently whispered to the new driver to go to the nearest hospital for humans so that we could end the whole nightmare in some sort of dignified fashion. During the entire ambulance ride, I continued the resuscitation effort. At this point the family had no idea how bad the injury had been. Every time I peered out of the ambulance's rear window I looked directly into the eyes of a hopeful Tracy Krosnoff, Jeff's wife.

The ambulance finally arrived at Toronto Western Hospital, located about three miles from the track. The attendants and I pushed Jeff into the emergency room, continuing to perform CPR (cardiopulmonary resuscitation). Jon Potter was already there. He had informed the hospital of what had happened and had begun to organize the family in a small room adjacent to the Emergency Department. I informed the not-too-happy ER physician who we were, what had happened, and how we had ended up in his place. Fortunately, he turned out to be very cooperative and pronounced Krosnoff dead without protest.

The coroner's office was notified and I went with Potter to inform the family. Needless to say his young wife took the news very badly. The parents were there as well, and they were also devastated. All of them were attending a CART race for the first time. Cal Wells, Jeff's car owner, was also very distraught. He and Krosnoff were very close friends. The last CART fatality had been in 1982, 14 years earlier. I was visibly shaken and felt the approaching signs of an impending anxiety attack.

About the time I was going to bolt for the Emergency Room door, I was jolted back into action. The media had already assembled across the street and was asking for a statement as to the driver's condition. At the same time, CART management was calling for information from the track, and the coroner had just arrived. Scully was on yet another phone, and the family needed my attention. My wife was calling from our medical unit, adding to the chaos. No time to get anxious. I had been up this road before and with Potter's help we managed to placate the press, talk to the family, inform the track and the CART officialdom, and to begin a detailed description of what had happened for the coroner and a police sergeant who accompanied him.

The acting coroner for the event in Toronto was a young emergency physician by the name of Trevor Gilmore. He arrived in the ER wearing white pants and a multi-colored Hawaiian shirt. He had been grilling steaks at home when the emergency call came. Potter instantly charmed the socks off Dr. Gilmore and we soon found out he liked racing as well as anything else associated with an element of danger. In addition to being the coroner and an emergency physician, he piloted a 747 for Air Canada in his spare time. He also performed rescue diving for the Canadian Coast Guard and was on Toronto's rapid response police squad (SWAT) team.

The police sergeant with Gilmore was referred to only as Fergie. He turned out to be a reasonable fellow as well. He tried to appear serious and tough, but deep down felt empathy for everyone involved. Both Dr. Gilmore and Fergie handled the session with professionalism and aplomb. The taped deposition took about two hours to complete. When we were done, Gilmore asked if he could join our Safety Team and Fergie suggested we all go someplace for a stiff drink.

The police released Krosnoff's body to the family the next day, unheard of when a death occurs in a foreign country. Dr. Scully was responsible for the smooth way in which the whole incident was handled by the local authorities. We arranged to follow up the investigation with Gilmore and Fergie at our Vancouver race in September. Potter and I were exhausted by this time and met Dr. Scully at Barberian's Steak House for several whiskeys and a good meal. It had been a long time since anything like this had happened and we were all still stunned.

After a long investigation, the Canadian government absolved CART of any wrongdoing. They declared Krosnoff's death a racing accident and made street-legal ambulances mandatory at all racing events in the province of Ontario. Gilmore did join the Safety Team as an alternate physician. Fergie attended several CART races as a guest and developed into quite a racing fan. The CART community eventually accepted the death as a rare, freak accident and the races continued uninterrupted. The tree Krosnoff hit was removed.

Sadly, a young corner worker had also been killed in the crash. He had worked the Toronto race for a number of years. He died when the right rear wheel of Krosnoff's car hit him, killing him instantly. His corner working partner, who was to look out for him, was also hit by debris and could not sound a proper warning due to her own injuries. It was the most tragic day for CART in 14 years of racing. We had once again been lulled into thinking the sport had become relatively safe.

The drivers, crews, medics, owners and spectators were all shocked back into the reality of death in sports. Automobile racing continues to be a dangerous activity, with death lying constantly in wait for the right opportunity. Cal Wells' team was one of the most safety-minded in the CART series. Wells continued to field a team for the remainder of the season but his zest for our form of racing was gone. After running Cristiano da Matta and Oriol Servià in 1999 and 2000, he would leave CART for the larger profits and exposure of NASCAR. He continues to work diligently to improve the safety of his drivers. He and his engineers have developed what is probably the safest seat in use in NASCAR today, setting an example for that series.

At first NASCAR turned it down thinking that it was too expensive and in some way might be a performance advantage for the Wells team. Due to persistence and the support of several drivers, the seat has now been fully accepted by NASCAR and is currently utilized by some of the top drivers. Automobile racing could use more owners like Cal Wells.

Chapter 26

EMERSON HAS
THE BIG ONE

Even though CART staged the US 500 at Michigan International Speedway in May, the annual Michigan 500 was scheduled, as usual, for late July 1996. Late July is prime vacation time in the upper Midwest and a reasonable crowd was expected for the race. Raceday was forecast to be hot and sunny, a tough event for the drivers since the race normally lasts for more than three hours. My wife and I arrived at the track early and you could already tell that the crowd was going to be huge. The first order of the day was breakfast at the Patrick Racing hospitality tent. Not only was it a good place to eat, you could also pick up on the latest racing gossip. Pat Patrick and Jack Bjerke, one of the CART attorneys, would usually be there, along with Wally Dallenbach, Al Speyer, head of Firestone Racing, and any number of other car owners who would saunter in and out looking for news and gossip. Talk would usually center on the plight of open-wheel racing in America.

After breakfast and a heated discussion as to how smart or dumb Tony George was, I ran into Emerson Fittipaldi standing outside the Penske Racing tent. We engaged in some casual conversation and I saw that familiar look in his eye. Hard to describe, it was a look of determination mixed with a little hostility. I was sure he was going to win the race. He was disappointed with his qualifying spot in the second row, but was very happy with his car following the final practice period. I told everyone in the medical unit that Emerson was going to win that day.

The race started under bright sunny skies, little wind, and the temperature near 90. Going into the second turn on the first lap, Emerson was charging for the lead trying to pass Greg Moore on the outside of the turn. He lost control of his car as he exited the turn. The car swapped ends and he crashed heavily into the outer retaining wall. The initial impact was to the left rear of the car, which burst into flames. Emerson later described a very eerie sensation. He told me that immediately after the impact he lost his color vision, everything appeared in various shades of black, white, and grey. He then felt himself being engulfed by the flames. He assumed he was going to die. All sound disappeared. He likely lapsed into momentary unconsciousness.

The next thing he described were noises gradually returning. First, he heard only a roaring sound then slowly he could discern the individual cars as they zoomed by. He happily realized the fire was gone and his color vision gradually returned to normal. The first person he recognized was Dr. Trammell. It was only then that he knew he would survive.

He tried to move his arms and legs and was relieved when everything worked. He described a tremendous pain in his chest and some difficulty getting a full breath. Trammell and I had learned from our crash studies that rear impacts were responsible for most of our neck fractures. Emerson was placed in a neck collar and a device called the 'Extricator' was used to stabilize his spine. This device is simply two parallel dowel rods supported by fabric and Velcro straps. When it is fastened properly it will restrain the thoracic and lumbar spine during the extrication process. With his spine immobilized, he was carefully removed from the car and placed in the ambulance for the trip to the medical center.

I had watched the crash as it occurred on the TV monitor located inside the medical unit. I was very concerned about the possibility of a neck fracture considering the magnitude and direction of the crash. Emerson arrived in the medical unit screaming to be let up off the stretcher.

"Steve, Sheet! Let me up! Let me go Steve, Sheet!" (Sheet is Brazilian for shit.)

"Please! Steve you are my friend, let me go!"

I was tempted to let him up, but I knew better. In spite of his constant pleading, I kept him on the spine board with his neck immobilized. He denied any pain in his neck, but complained bitterly about pain in his chest and lower back. His oxygen level was on the low side so I was also concerned about a collapsed lung. When I listened to his chest I could hear air moving on both sides and that told me that he was in no immediate danger, at least for the time being. Examining him further, I found a large bruise rapidly developing in his left flank. I decided to leave him as he was, started oxygen, and told the helicopter crew to get him to Foote Hospital in Jackson, Michigan as quickly as possible. Emerson was still yelling at me as the chopper took off for Jackson.

The race continued without any more serious incidents. About halfway into it, I received a call from the physician in Foote's Emergency Room. He reported that Emerson had a severe fracture of his seventh cervical vertebrae. He said that a bone fragment was lying next to the spinal chord and the chord was bent into an 'S' shape as a result. He also reported a partial collapse of his left lung and said that fluid was rapidly developing in the small of his back. The Mansell lesion! Like Nigel at Phoenix, the impact was so severe that shearing forces were tearing at his subcutaneous tissues. With a neck fracture of this type, had I allowed Emerson to get up off the backboard as he insisted, he would have been paralyzed forever from his neck down.

Foote Hospital was not the designated spine center for the area so they were required to move Emerson to the Regional Spine Center located in Kalamazoo, Michigan. When the race ended, Terry and I headed there.

In the ER we met the neurosurgeon assigned to Emerson's case. He was an older physician, very pleasant in his manner. He examined Emerson and told us his plans. He felt Emmo did not need surgery. He felt the injury could be treated conservatively with a halo vest, an externally applied contraption that immobilizes the head and neck, and bed rest for three months. The surgeon obviously didn't know much about Emerson. Putting Emerson to bed would be like trying to convince a shark to quit swimming.

Terry and I reviewed the films and felt that this was indeed a serious fracture that required extensive surgery, especially if Emerson was ever going to race again. We devised a plan and went to meet with Roger Penske.

In 1996 Lynne and I had been living in South Florida for five years. I had accepted a position at the University of Miami directing the Neuroscience Intensive Care Unit at Jackson Memorial Hospital, at the urging of an old classmate of mine, Dr. Barth Green. Dr. Green is a renowned neurospine surgeon and founder of the Miami Project to Cure Paralysis. Dr. Green is well respected internationally, and very well known in Miami. I called him from Michigan and explained what was going on with Emerson. Dr. Trammell spoke with Dr. Green in the language of spine surgeons and Dr. Green also agreed that Emerson needed surgery.

We could have taken Emerson to Indianapolis for the surgery but, since he lived in Miami and Dr. Green was keenly interested in the case, we elected to fly him home. I made sure that Terry would be allowed in the operating room and saw to it that Barth procured temporary staff privileges for Terry. Another advantage of going to Miami was that Emerson would end up in my Intensive Care Unit where I could keep a close eye on him following the surgery. Emerson could sell air conditioners to the Eskimos and needed strong supervision.

Surgery was scheduled for the next day. Again we were going to sign out of the hospital against medical advice. The local neurosurgeon thought we were all a little deranged. Explaining our plan to Emerson was easy, the hard part was telling Roger Penske that we were signing out against medical advice again and that we were going all the way to Miami for the surgery. Remembering Rick Mears, Penske accepted our plan and offered his jet for the flight. Terry would fly with Penske in his plane and I would accompany Emerson in a chartered hospital jet.

The chartered jet arrived for Emerson the next morning. We took off for Miami in our respective aircraft around 10 am. Emerson was in a lot of pain. I was giving him medication through a continuous intravenous line. He had a tube in his chest to protect his left lung, and had to remain with his neck immobilized in a very uncomfortable cocoon-like device used specifically for this kind of transport. He complained incessantly.

"Sheeet!"

The two jets flew in tandem and landed on schedule at Miami International Airport. We were met and taken by ambulance to Jackson Memorial Hospital for the surgery. Emerson's entire family was there by this time, as well as several of his friends. Emerson always had an entourage.

Dr. Green, Terry, and a local orthopedic spine surgeon named Frank Eismont operated on him for six hours. About halfway through the surgery there was, of all things, a bomb threat in the operating theater! The power went off and the generators kicked in. Good thing Emerson was asleep as we know he takes bomb threats quite seriously. Police were in and out of the operating room with the bomb-sniffing dogs. In spite of the interruption, the surgery went well. Emerson was transferred to my ICU about 11 o'clock that evening.

When he awakened, he realized how close he had come to being killed. He became very emotional and very thankful to be alive. Always the tough competitor, he was lapping the ICU with a walker in only two days. With his buttocks exposed he pushed his IV pole, urine bag attached, around the ICU with his hospital gown blowing in the wind.

He soon returned to his home on Key Biscayne and announced his retirement from professional racing a short time later. The surgeons had installed 16 screws and two plates in his neck and the risk of another accident with paralysis the likely result was simply too great. The crash had left him with a large collection of fluid almost identical to Mansell's. I drained the lesion daily in his home. During those visits we philosophized a lot over his phenomenal career and how lucky he was to have survived the sport's most dangerous years.

Emerson soon tackled his vast array of businesses, developing the same competitive urge he had demonstrated while racing. He dreamed of one day having his own team in CART, competing as an owner. Keeping him subdued while he recuperated was next to impossible. He was in the water exercising and riding his jet ski within a month. He was still the same old Emerson.

The computer reproduction of Emerson's crash demonstrated several inadequacies in the current level of cockpit protection. Ford Motor Company had designed the computer model with the information collected from our crash recorders. It was sophisticated enough to duplicate our crashes faithfully. With Ford's help we learned that Emerson's neck and head had been allowed to move about too freely in relation to his restrained torso. Using this valuable knowledge, we soon redesigned the head-surround area of the cockpit and the seat.

Extensive padding was placed over honeycomb material in the new head-surround structure. This new protection system afforded improved energy dissipation and limited the motion of both the head and neck, especially in a rear impact. Modifications of this basic head-surround structure are now used in Formula One, the IRL, and NASCAR. We were able to build the new system with a high degree of confidence based on knowledge from the computer simulations. The cars were now going even faster in the turns and often rotating less than 180 degrees before impact. Rear impacts were becoming the norm, especially on oval tracks.

The application of science to driver protection was developing rapidly. Terry and I were able to obtain videos of all of the crashes that produced an injury. We also had Dan Boyd, our own photographer, who obtained still photos of the damaged cars as well as photos of the accident scene. We personally inspected the wrecked cars, usually right after the crash. Crash recorder data was downloaded immediately by the Ford engineers and this information, coupled with the film and damage reports, soon led to better computer models. We were able to make changes to the cars, the seating position of the drivers, and the injury protection devices used, all without risking an actual driver in a crash as in the old trial-and-error method for change.

More and more information was forthcoming and a number of other improvements were made to the cockpit area as well as to the racecar itself. Seats were designed to fit the driver better and to support more fully the head, neck and torso. Sharp edges inside the cockpit were padded or eliminated. Padding for head injury protection was provided along the cockpit edges as far forward as driver comfort would allow. The front suspension was redesigned to impede intrusion of parts into the driver's compartment. Cockpit sides were elevated to support the shoulders better and to deflect errant parts ejected during a crash. Terry and I, along with the designers and engineers, thought we had finally developed a truly safe racecar. One that was capable of protecting our drivers in very high G impacts. In fact, we had drivers survive crashes as high as 145 G.

A lot of crashes occurred in 1997 and 1998, without any significant injuries. I was widely quoted in the media as to how safe our cars had become. Drivers were now retiring primarily due to age and not injury. New drivers fully expected to race until they were no longer competitive, expecting to retire gracefully and without disability. The atmosphere around the paddock was relaxed and almost partylike. The drivers remained fiercely competitive.

Chapter 27

OUR LUCK
RUNS OUT

Laguna Seca was probably CART's most picturesque venue. Nestled in the high, arid terrain outside of Carmel, California, the track weaves its way over the hills adjacent to old Fort Ord. The fort sprawls along the Pacific Coast isolating the track from the teeming crowds who live in or visit the area. When fog doesn't completely enshroud the place, you can see the entire Monterey coastline from the top of the Corkscrew, the famous left-right hand turn that descends five stories into the valley below. Everyone loved to go to Laguna.

Saturday morning practice for the 1999 race was delayed for over two hours because of drizzle and fog, not an unusual occurrence at Laguna Seca in the Fall. The rescue helicopter was unable to fly due to the limited visibility, but I had just informed Wally Dallenbach that the fog had lifted sufficiently for an ambulance to travel safely. As far as I was concerned, it was safe to start the practice session. The Chief Steward agreed. The announcement was made for the teams to get ready and Terry put on his firesuit. He grabbed his latest spy novel and joined Dave Hollander in Safety 2. In 18 years we had never seriously hurt anyone at Laguna and Terry and I were looking ahead to dinner that evening at Casanova's famous Italian restaurant in Carmel.

In the Penske pit Rick Mears was advising their new driver, Gonzalo Rodriguez, about how to go fast on this particular track. Rodriguez, aged 23, was from Uruguay. It was his first day to drive what we now had to call a Champ Car. Mears was now working as a consultant to Penske's team, hired to work with its drivers as a mentor, advocate, and father figure. Rodriguez was new to

CART racing and had a lot to learn. He had looked good in some smaller series such as Formula 3000 in Europe, but had yet to prove himself in the big cars. The fog lifted a bit as the green flag was waived to begin practice.

I was stuck in the med center as usual but didn't really mind. The day was damp and cold, I would just as soon be inside.

"Yellow! Yellow! Yellow!" soon came over the safety channel.

I quickly glanced at the TV monitor. All I saw was a view of the retaining wall just beyond the top of the Corkscrew. A severely torn advertising banner was flapping in the breeze. There was nothing else on the screen. Soon, a Safety Truck arrived at the scene and the guys jumped out and headed for the wall. Terry was in that truck. I watched as he slipped then fell while running frantically to the scene. I couldn't understand why they were all in such a hurry. Then they showed it. From a different camera angle, a racecar was seen on the other side of the wall, upside down, flat as a pancake against the earth. It was several feet down the steep embankment. A photographer standing nearby rushed over to the car, looked down, then abruptly turned and ran away.

Terry stumbled again as he cleared the wall. He raced down the hill towards the car. Some of the other safety guys had already reached the crash site. It did not look good.

"Steve, it's a Code 10!"

I couldn't believe it. The car looked as if it had only sustained some minor damage. Looking closely at a view of the impact point, now being shown on the TV, I was able to make out a large splash of red, exactly where the car had gone over. It was blood, not paint. I learned later from Terry that Rodriguez had bled out completely before the car ever hit the ground. His entire blood volume was on the wall, the banner, and the ground leading up to the car.

Accident reconstruction would show that Rodriguez had hit the wall in a slightly nose-down attitude after becoming airborne when he left the pavement. This caused his torso to be ejected upward and forward out of the seat. This motion was stopped by the shoulder belts as his head continued to accelerate unhindered from his body. His skull separated from his vertebral column, severing the large blood vessels that supply the brain. The hemorrhage from his nose and mouth was massive. Death was instantaneous.

We were stunned! Shocked in disbelief! My attention turned to the radio. While loading Rodriguez into the ambulance, an altercation had suddenly erupted. I overheard the ambulance crew inform Terry that since he had declared the driver dead he could not move him from the crash site. Thankfully, reason soon prevailed and the body was taken to the Community Hospital of the Monterey Peninsula to be properly pronounced.

Some of our safety guys were new and had never seen anything like it. They wandered around in a daze. Potter, Father Phil, and I left for the hospital immediately. The Penske entourage with Roger himself followed close behind.

In the emergency room, Rodriguez's body looked as if he had simply gone to sleep. There were no visible signs of injury. A very handsome boy, the sight was macabre. Not a mark anywhere. No one from his family was at the race. He had come to America alone to race for Roger Penske.

Road racing in CART was thought to be relatively safe with little risk of serious injury. Jeff Krosnoff's death in '96 was considered a fluke, and no one had died for 14 years before that. The entire CART contingent was thrown into a state of disbelief and anger. The drivers were especially upset and asked for an immediate meeting with the CART officials. They needed to ventilate before they could face driving at speed again.

Roger Penske and I notified the family in Uruguay via cell phone. Father Phil interpreted for them as they spoke only Spanish. I felt for them greatly. The coroner arranged for the body to be flown to Uruguay the next day. Penske and Father Phil also went to be with the family, and attended the funeral. Terry and I started our investigation into the crash to see what had gone wrong.

The consensus was that Rodriguez had entered the turn too

fast. When he tried to slow down, he locked up the front wheels braking too hard. Some theorized that he may have caught his foot between the throttle and brake pedal as he tried to panic stop. This would cause the car to continue accelerating until it left the course. He became airborne when the pavement changed to gravel. When he hit the wall, the nose-down angle of impact caused the car to catapult over not only the wall, but also the advertising banner hanging high above it. Had he hit the wall head-on in a level attitude, his head would likely have hit the padded steering wheel, resulting in a concussion but nothing more. This was the first basilar skull fracture to occur in the CART series.

Terry and I had dinner as planned in Carmel. Although more subdued, we still managed to laugh a little and enjoyed a good bottle of wine. Racing was still dangerous and we were comfortable that it was driver error that caused the death. We didn't know Rodriguez beforehand, but we felt very sad for his family back home. We went to bed feeling secure that this was an isolated occurrence and not likely to happen again.

Three weeks after the Laguna Seca tragedy we found ourselves in California again for the 500-mile race in Fontana. The glistening California Speedway is a high-speed, two-mile, super speedway. It is the fastest open-wheel race track in the world. Brazilian driver Mauricio Gugelmin set the closed course record of 240.942 mph there while setting pole position in 1997. Like Michigan, I always brought a third physician to Fontana. The California Speedway could rapidly become a very busy race track. Dr. Jay Phelan, previously from California and still licensed there, was the customary choice.

Practice for the race had gone extremely well, with no significant crashes. It was the end of the season and everyone was in a festive mood. Several end-of-the-year parties were planned for Sunday and Monday, and most of us were looking forward to some time away from traveling. Canadian Greg Moore was no exception. He had not had the season he and everyone else had expected. A number of bone-headed moves had caused him to crash out early from several events. Everyone knew he held a ton of promise. In fact, Roger Penske had already signed him to drive for his team in 2000. At Fontana the weekend was going better than expected. Greg was running with the fastest guys in practice and was anticipating a start well up in the field.

As qualifying was about to begin on Saturday, Moore was riding through the paddock on his familiar light blue scooter, joking with friends, and signing autographs for his many fans. As he made a turn into the parking area, a lady in a passenger car abruptly pulled out in front of him. Moore could not avoid the crash. He was thrown from his scooter, breaking the little finger of his right hand. The lady felt horrible, but Moore felt a lot worse. His plans for a good race were now in serious jeopardy. He had the contract with Penske for 2000, and wanted to finish on a high note for the Player's organization which had sponsored him up to that point.

Moore came to the medical center with his father Ric and a representative from the Player's team. Greg's dad did all of the talking.

"He can race can't he, tell me he can race?"

"We'll have to see", I said. "Dr. Trammell needs to take a look at this."

I called Terry to the unit and we X-rayed the obviously broken finger. The break was bad, but Terry said it could be splinted temporarily and fixed permanently at a later date. If the pain was bearable, we both felt he could race safely.

The scooter crash had caused Moore to miss qualifying. A short test was needed to evaluate whether he could drive safely with the splint. The rules stated that he would have to start in the back of the field.

The test was arranged for the end of the day. Greg would run several laps under observation by the stewards following the last practice session. A special pair of gloves would be needed to accommodate his swollen and splinted finger. His team quickly manufactured a unique four-fingered glove, with one very large finger to accommodate the injured digit and the one next to it.

Moore pulled on to the track under the watchful eyes of Dr. Trammell, the Chief Steward, and me. As Director of Medical Affairs, I was ultimately responsible for a driver's return to competition. For orthopedic injuries I always took Terry's advice, but it was still my ultimate responsibility. Greg quickly got up to speed. He executed a series of laps that would have placed him on the front row for the race. After a brief discussion, we cleared him to race. Telemetry from the car's data recorder showed he had used the steering wheel perfectly during the test. There was some minor grumbling among some of the drivers and opposing team members, but nearly everyone was happy to have Greg in the race. His father was especially happy. Ric Moore thanked Terry and me again and again.

Raceday dawned California bright and sunny. A near sellout crowd was on hand, with the infield packed. As the drivers approached their cars for the pre-race ceremonies Greg told his friends Max Papis, Paul Tracy, and Jimmy Vasser:

"I'll see you up front!"

The race started on schedule. Moore immediately began passing cars. He chose the outside line around Turns 1 and 2, running very close to the wall. He was passing cars at will, on his way to the front as promised. On lap 34, Richie Hearn lost control of his car high in Turn 2. He spun wildly into the infield grass, heading straight toward the inside retaining wall. He hit the wall hard with the left front of the car, sliding along it for a few feet. The impact angle was approximately 45 degrees. The car was badly damaged, but Hearn climbed out of it unhurt. He was taken by ambulance to our medical center for an examination and observation. He was subsequently released with only a bruised ego.

The green light went back on while Hearn was still socializing in the medical center. He was watching the TV monitor with the nurses and remarked how fast Moore was driving. Greg had already reached ninth place and was in a wheel-to-wheel duel with five other cars. While Hearn was discussing how scary it looked, Moore lost control of his car on the outside of Turn 2 in an attempt to pass three cars in one heroic move. The back of his car jumped to the right and he headed straight for the infield grass. He did not spin as Hearn had. Instead, he vaulted from the track at over 200 mph, becoming airborne as the surface changed from asphalt to grass. He soared for a distance of over 30 yards before landing hard on the left front wheel. The impact dug a large divot in the infield. The car somehow remained upright but was tilted severely to the left. It then plowed into the same wall that Hearn had hit at roughly the same angle but with a much higher velocity. The two drivers had impacted the wall within 30 feet of each other.

The result of Moore's impact was an immediate disintegration of the car followed by a series of violent side-over-side flips and further destruction. Greg's arms could be seen flailing wildly outside the cockpit as the car rolled over and over. He finally came to rest upside down, more than 100 feet from the original impact site.

The nurses and I watched a replay of the crash inside the medical unit while the Safety Trucks rushed to the scene. It was several minutes before Terry's report came over our private channel.

"I don't think he's gonna make it! I'm coming in with him."

I told Terry to go straight to the helicopter, I would meet him there. It was stationed inside the medical compound just outside of our medical unit. Soon several people rushed the security guard at the gate. Included were media representatives, fans, and assorted others intent on seeing the well-liked driver. Jon Potter, with the help of Greg Passauer, driver of our medical unit and designated bouncer, soon had the crowd under reasonable control with the help of local security.

Terry arrived with Moore in the ambulance. He and one of the local paramedics were attempting to breathe for him using an oxygen bag and mask. They had tried unsuccessfully to place a tube in his airway while *en route*. This had been impossible due to the jostling and relative darkness inside the speeding ambulance. Moore was in near cardiac arrest when he arrived at the heliport.

One of the other paramedics and I quickly placed a breathing tube in his trachea and cardiopulmonary resuscitation was started. His heartbeat was undetectable, with a chaotic heart rhythm visible on the cardiac monitor. His head had assumed a grotesque appearance, being purple in color and very swollen. The pupils of his eyes were fixed and dilated with the empty stare that accompanies a severe head injury. Moore was near death. We placed him in the helicopter with the med-evac squad continuing to do CPR. TV was waiting for a live report. I gave the following statement:

"Greg Moore has been severely injured with massive head injuries and multiple fractures. He is being air lifted to Loma Linda Hospital where further resuscitative measures will be undertaken."

My message contained the unmistakable hint of death. My hands were shaking and I could feel my voice quiver as I spoke. I was feeling the familiar pangs of anxiety. Andrew Craig, CEO of CART at the time, notified me that there was to be a press conference immediately after the race. I walked back to the unit and as soon as I walked through the door the call came in from Loma Linda. Moore was dead. The doctors there had tried unsuccessfully to resuscitate him for more than 25 minutes. They had even opened his chest hoping to find a treatable injury. There was none. Moore's body and head had been virtually destroyed in the crash.

I joined the nurses who were hugging each other and crying uncontrollably. Everybody loved Greg Moore. He became an instant friend to everyone he met. He had no enemies. He was characteristically charging to the very end. That was how Greg Moore drove. Telemetry would show that he had continued to drive his car until he hit the wall. He had the throttle floored as he left the track. That's why he went airborne. He was actually accelerating, trying to regain control of the car. He continued to steer it while he was hurtling across the grass. His steering input, up until the time he crashed, had been precise. He never gave up, not until the end.

The press conference was held. It was the most difficult I had ever been in. The media of course wanted to know if his broken finger had played a role in the crash. I assured them that it did not. They asked a lot of questions I didn't have the answers to. Some people who watched the race on television later told me they could tell from my expression during the announcement that Greg was dead.

All the year-end parties scheduled that night were cancelled. Terry was really distraught. He walked aimlessly around the garage area for some time after the race. He was looking for answers. There was nothing to second guess. The injuries were non-survivable. There was nothing that could have been done that would have saved his life. CART had lost a great driver, a true friend, and a remarkable personality. Greg's memory lives on to this day. He will never be forgotten by any of us who knew him, who raced against him, or who simply watched him.

The day after the accident Wally Dallenbach and I, and the rest of the key officials, went back to the scene of the crash to get a better understanding of what had happened, as well as what may have caused the various injuries. Moore's impact was only a few feet from that of Richie Hearn. If only Greg had spun the car and hit the brake instead of choosing the throttle, he would likely have had the same crash as Hearn. We reminded ourselves that what ifs don't help. We inspected the wrecked car, going over every square inch. The result of our own inquest offered no surprises. The car did its job as well as it could considering the magnitude of the crash. The wheel tethers, added earlier in the year to keep wheels and tires from becoming missiles, did their job. The front wheels and tires did not cause any of Greg's injuries. The rollover hoop was intact. Greg, in his quest to get up front, was betrayed by the sudden transition from asphalt to grass. The transition, at the speed he was traveling, caused sufficient air to flow under his front wing that he became airborne. This hazardous design was changed as a result of the crashes at both Fontana and Michigan. The grassy areas were paved, making the chance of becoming airborne much less likely. Sadly, it often takes a tragic crash to reveal a potentially deadly situation.

Chapter 28

LOOKING FOR ANSWERS AND THE COMING OF HANS

In the fall of 1999, Dr. Trammell and I were preparing our presentations for the annual meeting of the International Council of Motorsports Sciences to be held in London. This was the first time the ICMS would meet jointly with the Medical Commission of the Fédération Internationale de l'Automobile (FIA). The ICMS is an organization that arose following a meeting held in 1985 that included Dr. Trammell and I, along with Dr. Dan Marisi and Dr. Jacques Dallaire, both from McGill University. The four of us met in the bar of the Hilton Hotel in downtown Indianapolis following the 500 Mile race. Jacques and Dan had been testing the fitness of Formula One drivers and other elite athletes for a couple of years in Canada. They studied the physical and mental attributes of a competitive racing driver and what sets the good ones apart from those who are not so good. Jacques and Dan were both exercise physiologists, with Dan having a second doctorate in sports psychology. Each of them had a keen interest in what constitutes a successful racing driver.

Because Terry and I had the same interests, the four of us became acquainted when our paths inevitably crossed at the Speedway. Jacques and Dan were helping Canadian driver Jacques Villeneuve with his training and fitness program and as such were frequent visitors in the garage area. Informal discussions among the four of us were growing more numerous and we decided to have dinner at some point over race weekend.

As we were enjoying cocktails before dinner, I voiced the opinion that we probably weren't the only scientists interested in racecar drivers. There were likely several professionals scattered throughout the world either observing, or actually studying, the effects of motorsport on the human body. The others agreed.

We kept in touch over the remainder of the year and succeeded in forming a fledgling council after sending inquiries to the few people we knew that might be interested. By the spring of 1986, our collective efforts had garnered nearly 30 members. The inaugural meeting of the new organization was set for May in Indianapolis, exactly one year after our cocktails at the Hilton.

That first meeting was held in a small auditorium at Methodist Hospital. The program consisted of mostly anecdotal stories of each other's experiences with some spectacular crash pictures thrown in. Although there were few, if any, real scientific studies presented, a great deal of positive energy was generated from the meeting. We adjourned with the charge of finding new members for the following year and encouraging current members to submit papers.

By 1999, 14 years later, membership had grown to more than 140. Representation included delegates from 11 different countries. Most of the members were physicians, but there was a sizable contingent of nurses, paramedics, athletic trainers, exercise physiologists, and biomechanical engineers. The meetings had advanced in stature and now included a number of valid scientific papers. The organization gained most of its early credibility from the data that Terry and I generated with our crash recorders.

The information we presented had tweaked the interest of Dr. John Melvin and Dr. Jim Lighthall from General Motors, Dr. Robert Hubbard from Michigan State University, Dr. Pria Prasad from Ford Motor Company, Dr. Ted Knox from Wright-Patterson Air Force Base, Dr. Richard Jennings from NASA, Dr. Hubert Gramling from Daimler-Chrysler, Dr. Andy Mellor from TRL (the UK's Transport Research Laboratory), and several other well-known crash and injury investigators. As the meetings progressed, these scientists began to work collegially on improving safety and performance within the sport. As the organization's initial chairman, I tried to encourage this cooperation.

Several independent projects were soon undertaken at various locations throughout the world. With Dr. Lighthall, an exercise physiologist, I attempted to settle the question of whether or not a racing driver is an athlete by designing a study to monitor heart rate during competition. Dr. Trammell analyzed crash recorder data together with Dr. Melvin, the better to understand the mechanisms for spine and extremity injuries. Dr. Hubbard developed his now famous HANS device with his brother-in-law Jim Downing during this same period. Dr. Prasad worked on improving computer simulations of crashes and Dr. Mellor and Dr. Gramling developed improvements in the Formula One cars. That 14-year period was the true renaissance period for motorsports safety.

Toronto's Dr. Hugh Scully became chairman of the ICMS in 1998. I continued on the Board of Directors while Jon Potter served as the organization's Executive Secretary. Scully was a longtime friend of Professor Sid Watkins, the Medical Delegate for Formula One and founder and head of the FIA's esteemed Medical Commission. Scully thought the time was right for a joint meeting of the FIA and the ICMS. Potter, Scully, and I began to plan such a meeting. Scully presented the plan to Professor Watkins who accepted it without reservation. The first joint meeting of the two organizations was scheduled for mid-winter in London.

By meeting jointly, we were able to share information with a new group of scientists and professionals from Europe. Even NASCAR was represented with the appearance of Dave Holcomb, their risk manager. Never interested before, NASCAR got wind of the meeting and felt they should be represented. Instead of sending a physician or nurse, they sent their risk manager. NASCAR had never had a Medical Director and had always left safety in the hands of the participants and the race tracks. Holcomb would eventually become a board member of ICMS and NASCAR's representation and interest within the organization would increase in the future.

The ICMS is now well established with valid research ongoing.

Improvements in the provision of on-track care, drivers' personal equipment, in-car protection, safety at the race tracks themselves, and spectator safety have all benefited from the efforts of the members and their various research projects. Examples of these cooperative efforts include but are not limited to: the development of improved head and neck protection in the cockpit with a newly designed head-surround system; improvement of seatbelts and their anchor points; improvement in car integrity and design; better methods for the extrication and initial treatment of drivers; improved in-car seating; and the development and implementation of the HANS device worldwide.

Dr. Robert Hubbard presented his HANS device at that winter meeting in London. He had presented it for the first time years earlier, but it was impractical for open-wheel cars due to its size and configuration. HANS simply stands for Head And Neck Support. It's a collar-shaped device with a yoke arrangement that fits over the driver's shoulders. The collar extends upward behind the neck and contains a tether on each side that attaches to the helmet. The HANS is anchored in the car by the driver's shoulder belts. It is made from lightweight composite materials. With the HANS in place the head, neck and thorax all move in the same direction during a crash.

The device appears deceptively simple. Refinement took more than 13 years. Mario Andretti tried it during a tire test sometime in the mid-80s and found it to be unbearable. Hubbard doggedly stuck with his design. He eventually presented the device to Dr. Melvin at Wayne State University in the late 80s. Melvin studied it in his laboratory and showed that, on dummies at least, neck loads in a crash were decreased anywhere from 40 to 60%. Jim Downing, Hubbard's brother-in-law who actually thought of the device, used the HANS faithfully when he raced his sportscar. For a long time he was the only one.

The HANS device smoldered along for a number of years with only a few drivers following Downing's lead and using it in sportscar competition. Definitive testing of it had not yet been accomplished. That would soon change, however. In 1994 a massive tragedy befell Formula One. Two drivers were killed on the same weekend at the San Marino Grand Prix. On the Saturday, Austrian rookie Roland Ratzenberger died in a heavy impact. The following day the sport's reigning superstar, Ayrton Senna, was also killed. After his death, which was captured on TV, the FIA launched an intensive investigation into the cause. Senna's head injuries were substantial. A piece of suspension had reportedly penetrated his visor and lodged in his brain. He had also smashed one side of his head against the concrete retaining wall where the crash occurred in the Tamburello corner. The investigation determined a need to improve the in-car protection of the driver's head and neck; the same goal we were pursuing in CART at the time due to fellow Brazilian Emerson Fittipaldi's crash in Michigan.

Tests were soon launched at Daimler-Chrysler under the direction of Dr. Hubert Gramling to see if airbags had any use in racecars. During these tests, a colleague of Dr. Gramling, mostly out of curiosity, offered a HANS device to compare it to the airbags. To everyone's surprise the HANS outperformed the airbags in every type of simulated crash. Armed with this information, Gramling began a concerted effort to develop the HANS further in order to make it more user-friendly. He and Hubbard worked closely together to refine it for potential open-wheel use.

The end result was a new, composite HANS, lighter in weight, much smaller, and less obtrusive. What happened next would revolutionize safety in motorsports, but I'm getting ahead of the story. Suffice it to say that the newly designed HANS performed well in laboratory crashes using high-speed sleds and dummies. Gramling and Hubbard presented their findings at the London meeting. Terry and I were very impressed by these results and started to push the HANS within CART.

We asked our colleagues at Ford to apply Gramling's data to a simulation of the Rodriguez crash at Laguna Seca. The Ford engineers determined that, had Rodriguez been wearing a HANS, he would have likely survived the crash. With this new bit of information in hand, I invited Dr. Hubbard to present the device to our drivers at the start of the 2000 season. Dr. Trammell, a graduate engineer as well as a physician, was convinced the HANS would be the future for neck protection in a racecar.

Hubbard's presentation to the drivers was generally well received although there were a few skeptics. Following the meeting, I met with one of the biggest, Christian Fittipaldi. Emerson's high-strung nephew was one of the pickiest drivers in the whole lot. He needed to have everything in his car, and on himself, just so. Most Brazilian drivers are picky about their creature comforts, but Christian topped the list. He was also a good friend of mine so I was able to convince him to be the guinea pig for the HANS.

When we started the project, he was driving for the Newman-Haas team. Fittipaldi generously devoted his entire winter test season to HANS development. Hubbard worked closely with the team and by the time the season rolled around Fittipaldi was ready to wear the device in competition. If he was comfortable with the device, I knew we could eventually make all of the drivers comfortable. I pushed CART to make the HANS mandatory for oval tracks in 2001. I strongly encouraged its use on road courses as well. Dr. Trammell was in total agreement. We were the first motorsports organization to mandate the HANS. Several lives have been saved and many injuries have been prevented since its implementation. The racing world owes a large debt of gratitude to Bob Hubbard and Jim Downing for their marvelous invention.

Chapter 29

THE DRIVER

AS ATHLETE

From 1990 through 2000, safety in motorsports improved markedly. Much of the improvement was a direct result of the ICMS and FIA membership getting together with the automobile manufacturers to push research and development. Along with these increased safety initiatives there was renewed interest in the physiological aspects of driving a racecar. Fierce competition, developing in all major series, was making it apparent that drivers needed to be physically fit in order to be competitive. At practically every race I attended, I was asked the same question:

"Are race drivers really athletes?"

I knew they were, but it was hard to convince others. I was determined to settle the issue once and for all. Most of the general public, and scientists as well, could not conceive of a driver being an athlete. They equated driving a racecar with driving their personal car. There is no comparison. In 1994, Dr. Jim Lighthall and I published a paper describing the heart rate responses to driving an open-wheeled racecar in competition. We undertook the study for two reasons. One, we felt strongly that drivers were being neglected by the sport's medicine community and, two I needed scientific data to back up my comments to the press.

Our study showed that drivers developed heart rates in the range of 80 to 85% of their maximum heart rate in response to the rigors of competitive driving. This did not surprise us, but it did shock a lot of disbelievers. How could driving a racecar be that physically demanding? I presented the paper at the ICMS meeting in Paris in 1994. I was told by a French scientist at the conclusion of my talk that the high heart rates were the result of anxiety and apprehension and not physical effort. In other words, this guy was convinced the high heart rates were due to adrenalin, the result of fear, and not exertion. Even though we showed that the high heart rates dropped quickly to normal during caution periods, he still thought the high rates were due to fear. It would be another eight years before it could be shown once and for all that race drivers utilize oxygen to the same degree that many other traditional athletes do in competition.

Drivers also exhibit other athletic attributes. Dr. Dan Marisi had shown years earlier that drivers not only require tremendous hand, eye, and foot coordination, they also require the ability to sort through what is taking place in front of, and around them, at any given moment. Sports opthalmologists have shown that racing drivers have an increased awareness of what is in their visual field. All of us have roughly the same visual field, but not all of us are keenly aware of everything within that field. Tests have shown that professional racing drivers have the same visual field capabilities as professional football quarterbacks and hockey and soccer goalies.

Drivers must also have the ability to anticipate events far in advance of them actually happening. This should come as no surprise since, as alluded to earlier, racecars travel more than the length of a soccer field every second at 200 mph. Just as a quarterback must instantly be able to assess the best option available to gain yards, so must a racing driver be able to discern the best path to take to get to the front of the pack or to avoid a crash.

In 2002, together with Dr. Pat Jacobs, an exercise physiologist at the Miami Project to Cure Paralysis, I utilized a new portable device that could actually measure the amount of oxygen consumed during a sporting activity. Previously, an athlete always had to be attached to a huge metabolic monitor roughly the size of a washing machine while running on either a treadmill or riding a bicycle, to determine his or her maximum oxygen consumption (VO_2 max). Now, thanks to miniaturization, we can measure VO_2 max with a device called the KDR-2. This is roughly the size of a

VHS cassette tape. It can easily be attached to the driver's torso using Velcro. Tubes run from the device to a special oxygen mask cleverly fitted to a standard racing helmet. The whole apparatus fits into the cockpit of a modern racecar without interfering with the driver's ability to drive.

I convinced Mauricio Gugelmin to use the device during an off-season test in Sebring, Florida. Dr. Jacobs and I found in that initial test that drivers utilize oxygen at the rate of 12 to 13 METs (metabolic equivalents). One MET is the amount of energy required simply to sit still. Thirteen METs is roughly equivalent to singles tennis at the professional level, swimming 1,500 meters at the Olympics, or the pace required in a full marathon. Prior to the test, Dr. Jacobs was very skeptical. He became a believer as soon as Gugelmin's results were tabulated. In an automobile race, there are no timeouts. Pit stops last only 12 to 15 seconds. Drivers are performing at this high level of energy expenditure for anywhere from two to four hours. Are drivers athletes? You bet they are.

This level of exertion is in response to the high longitudinal and lateral G-forces generated by the cars as they negotiate corners, accelerate, and brake. With modern tires and suspension systems, as stated before, lateral Gs can exceed five in tight, high-speed corners. With a three-pound helmet, it is the equivalent of having a 15-pound weight tied to your head that is constantly swinging to and fro. A second study, using the same apparatus, showed that road courses are nearly twice as physically demanding as ovals. Yes, drivers are athletes and no, you can't successfully compete in the major forms of automobile racing unless you are aerobically fit and physically and mentally quite strong.

Chapter 30

Ongoing Research and Development

D r. Trammell and I began to devote most of our time to the study of injury prevention. He investigates all of the orthopedic injuries and has become the world authority on the use of the HANS device. I investigate the causes and effects of head injury. We work in concert, and share data on nearly a daily basis. Terry has been able to use the information he gathers to perform better as a spine and orthopedic surgeon in Indianapolis while I have been able to do the same with treating head- and spine-injured patients in Miami.

The 'Magician' has operated on more than 90% of the drivers at one time or another. His combination of engineering and medical skills enables him to tailor his orthopedic care to the injury at hand. The injuries he faces are usually not simple, but are often very complex and require imagination and guts to repair. The best example is that of Rick Mears but there have been many others. Textbooks don't describe these kinds of injuries because they are unique. By employing artful reconstructive skills, Trammell can often return drivers to competition much sooner than expected. He is revered by the drivers, their teams, and their families.

Usually, if a bone is broken you can realign it, immobilize it and then wait for it to heal. If you have pneumonia you find the right antibiotic and treat it. If an appendix is inflamed and about to rupture, you remove it. The care and treatment of a brain-injured patient, however, is not so precise. To date, very little is known about the actual forces and mechanisms involved in the generation of most head injuries. What information we do have comes from animal, cadaver, mannequin and computer models. Animal and cadaver brains are very different from living human brains. Most animal studies are based around a single impact to the brain. That is not what happens in a typical crash. We have learned that the head bounces around all over the place, being subjected to accelerations in virtually every direction. Often, the head doesn't hit anything at all as in the Rodriguez crash, yet the resulting injury can be catastrophic.

Several good computer models for head injury have been developed using clinical data as well as information gained from the various cadaver, animal and dummy tests. These models, however, lack real-time data and they are based on inferred information, not necessarily what really happens. There is a definite need to find a better way to analyze head injury as it unfolds.

Concussion, an injury to the brain that does not cause detectable structural damage but may have long-lasting effects on the victim, is also poorly understood. The case of National Football League quarterback, Steve Young, and his forced retirement from football illustrates this point well. Too many minor brain injuries too close together can have a cumulative effect over time, leading to poor judgment, altered reflexes, dementia and adverse effects on daily living, especially as one grows older.

In the winter of 1999, I arranged a meeting in Sebring, Florida to evaluate an idea I had that would allow head injury to be studied in a different way than ever before. I invited representatives from Endevco Corporation, a company that makes accelerometers for industrial use. Accelerometers measure the direction and magnitude of forces acting on an object. I also invited John Melvin, Ted Knox and representatives from Ford. I invited Doug Hill from Trice Motorsports Research who held a CRADA (Cooperative Research And Development Agreement) with the military and a representative from Motorola Racing Radios. A CRADA allows private concerns to interract and share data with the military. Racing Radios supplies the in-helmet radios for all of the CART teams as well as most other racing series.

In the meeting, I introduced the concept of using the driver's earpieces as a type of crash recorder for the head. The earpieces allow the drivers to communicate with their crews. They are held in place by the helmet and in over 25 years of attending crashes I have never seen an earpiece become dislodged. I reasoned that if accelerometers could be made small enough to fit into the earpieces, and they didn't bother the driver, we might be able to measure and record the forces directed against the head during a crash. The system, if it could be developed, must not interfere with the driver's ability to perform, or his ability to receive accurate information from his team. The data obtained had to be highly accurate and reproducible.

When I finished my presentation in Sebring, the assembled group looked at me as if I were nuts. A two-hour discussion ensued and the more the idea was discussed the more intrigued the participants became. We adjourned late in the afternoon and everyone went back to their laboratories to see if the concept was at all feasible. Several weeks later reports began to filter into my office in Miami.

Endevco had decided that they were able to develop a tiny, tri-axial accelerometer that would fit into the earpieces. Racing Radios had figured out how to assemble a system to house the accelerometers and still meet all of the communication needs. Dr. Knox and Dr. Melvin thought it might just work, but they remained somewhat dubious.

A second meeting was held at the Miami Project offices to set a timetable for development. I was thrilled. Maybe I wasn't crazy after all! John Melvin and Ted Knox began testing prototypes at Wayne State University and Wright-Patterson AFB respectively in the winter of 2000. Melvin was able to join a study funded by the FBI to evaluate the efficacy and safety of rubber bullets for riot control. He placed the earpiece system in the ear canal of the FBI cadaver and then hit its helmeted head with a rubber mallet. The device worked! It recorded an impact of over 100 Gs. Knox meanwhile tested the device in a crash dummy in his lab at Wright-Patterson. He also obtained reproducible results. It was soon time to take the ear accelerometers into the field.

The first field test of the new apparatus was held at Homestead Miami Speedway. Dr. Knox simply placed the device in an Indycar and started the engine. It was statically advanced to full throttle. The device again functioned well. There was no significant interference from the engine's electronics. Next, Knox took the device to the Mid-Ohio race track for a test in a Skip Barber Dodge car using their test driver as a guinea pig. For the first time, we were able directly to measure the direction, as well as the magnitude, of the forces the head is subjected to by simply driving the car. The head actually bounces around considerably as the driver negotiates the course.

Deep into the ear canal is about as close to the brain as we can get without directly entering the skull. Forces measured there represent the motion of the skull as long as the earpiece fits snugly. Sadly, Endevco lost interest in the project. In retrospect, I think they felt that there was little in the way of market potential for the device since the use was confined to a relatively small group of athletes. Most of us in the project thought they were markedly short-sighted. It is anticipated that information obtained from the ear accelerometers will be instrumental in developing improved helmets in a number of sports that require such head protection. Football, hockey and downhill skiing are three important ones.

Protective inner liners in helmets have not changed much in more than 30 years. Those of us who see athletic head injuries on a regular basis know that there must be a better way to build helmets. Good data is lacking, and helmet manufacturers are reluctant to change the current models for fear of liability. Head injury remains the biggest cause of death in all sports, not just racing. Data obtained from the ear accelerometer systems over the next several years should help engineers design improved testing standards for helmets. It is entirely conceivable that a coach on the sidelines will one day be able instantly to pull an athlete out of the game if he has sustained a blow to his head that exceeds a pre-determined concussion threshold.

When Endevco dropped out of the program, development of the device slowed. Mauricio Gugelmin had experimented with the system in one of the CART races with moderately successful results. The installation was difficult and he wasn't happy with the fit. It was also difficult to download the data from the car at the end of practice without hampering the team. The original accelerometer was still too large to fit into the earpiece as close to the brain as we wanted it.

Delphi Automotive Systems, in Vandalia, Ohio, close to Wright-Patterson AFB came to the rescue. They were sponsoring a car in the rival Indy Racing League at the time and, after learning about the earpiece accelerometers from Dr. Knox, felt there was potential for the device as well as a potential market. Their researchers went to work and quickly designed a smaller, more versatile accelerometer. They were able to place this version further into the earpiece. Additionally, they cleaned up the entire system so that it was better integrated with the rest of the electronics and more user-friendly for the driver and crew. We were back on track.

By 2002 the new Delphi version was placed in three cars in the IRL and three cars in CART. Driver Scott Sharp in the IRL would have the only crash. A small one, but we obtained some accurate data. The system appeared so promising that Delphi provided both CART and the IRL with accelerometers for all of the drivers in 2003. Dr. Knox and I published a paper describing the original development of the system in the well-respected journal *Neurosurgery*. Everyone involved in the ear accelerometer project anticipates a wealth of data over the next several years.

Dr. Trammell and I, although not tired of the competition, were beginning to get as much enjoyment out of our research activities as we did going to the events. We felt that, along with others, we were leading a major assault on death and injury in motorsports. Interest in motorsports safety was exploding worldwide. Sanctioning bodies were cooperating with the automotive industry in an attempt to improve things. Even NASCAR was beginning to show an interest with increased presence at safety-related meetings. Trammell and I were looking forward to the future.

Chapter 31

CART Goes
to the Movies

In the spring of 2000, CART announced that Sylvester Stallone was going to produce and star in a movie about auto racing. Initially he was going to use Formula One as the backdrop for his story but dealing with Bernie Ecclestone and the rest of the Formula One executives proved to be too much of a hassle. Stallone ended the negotiations with them, and contacted CART. CART jumped at the chance. A deal was signed and the announcement was made at Homestead Miami Speedway.

I for one was thrilled. Since I was a boy I had wanted to have some involvement in a motion picture. No matter how small, I just wanted to be part of a major movie production. Around mid-August I was contacted by the production company and asked if I could fly to Montreal after our race in Laguna Seca to help film the movie's big crash scene. I answered with an emphatic yes! Lon Bromley was also asked to be in the scene, as well as old CART stalwart, Dave Hollander and newer medic, Cam Howie. Within 48 hours I had told everyone I knew.

September rolled around quickly and Lynne and I headed to Carmel for the race at Laguna. Shortly after we arrived, I began to feel sick. I was having periods of profuse sweating alternating with shaking chills. My body felt like I had been beaten with the proverbial rubber hose. I took my temperature and it was over 103! My budding film career was in serious jeopardy. I called the production company and told them to find someone else. They told me to hang in there, and maybe by Monday I would feel OK.

I spent the entire weekend inside the medical unit seeing only those patients truly needing a physician. By Sunday night, I felt no better. My temperature was still high. I was miserable! I told Lynne that I was going to cancel and fly straight back to Miami and go to bed.

"You're nuts! You'll never forgive yourself!"

She had a point. I called the production company and they informed me that I didn't really have to be in Montreal until Wednesday. The actual filming would not be done until then. I decided to go home on Monday as scheduled, and then fly to Montreal on Tuesday. My fever broke sometime during our flight home. I went straight to bed and slept most of the day on Tuesday. I left for Montreal on the evening flight feeling like you do after driving straight through to Florida from Indianapolis for Spring Break.

Warner Brothers put us up in a splendid hotel in the center of downtown Montreal. In addition to the four of us, Wally Dallenbach was also there. He had been hired as the technical advisor for the movie to make sure the race scenes weren't too outlandish. I went to bed still feeling poorly, hoping I could function well the next day. We were to be picked up in front of the hotel at 5:30 in the morning.

I awoke feeling halfway decent. I groggily made my way to the lobby to join up with the rest of the guys. They had been there since Monday and were going on and on about how cool the scene was going to be. The incident supposedly takes place on a rain-soaked track in Germany. Cristián de la Fuente, one of the stars, crashes in the rain, leaves the track airborne, then lands in a swollen river upside down and on fire. The car sets the surrounding woods on fire as it hurtles through the trees, and we, the fearless safety team, must rush through the flames and retrieve the injured driver, dragged to the river bank by Stallone and another driver in the race.

Bromley explained to me how the car used for the scene was actually an old wrecked CART tub. To get it into the river it was pulled over a launching ramp by a steel cable that ran through a pulley attached to a tow vehicle racing in the opposite direction. A dummy dressed to look like the actor rode helplessly inside the car as it sailed through the air.

Once the car flies through the woods and lands in the water, the real actor climbs into another tub that had been permanently anchored in the river. The second tub rotated around an anchored steel rod, allowing the actor to climb into the car and then be turned upside down like a barbequed pig. The actor then had to sit in the upturned car underwater until he is rescued by Stallone. To keep him alive while he's upside down, he is given compressed air by a diver using the buddy system of breathing. This all sounded too cool to me.

We were driven to the set by van where we met the First Assistant Director. He led us to the wardrobe trailer and told us to pick out our uniforms along with some waterproof underwear. We were going to be in and out of the river while constantly being drenched by rain for the better part of two days. Surprising to me, everyone connected with the film was very friendly and polite, and actually made us feel special.

Next, we were taken to the site of the BIG crash scene. There we met Rene Harlan, the director, and Sylvestor Stallone the star. Beyond cool! Dallenbach was already there, sitting in a chair with his name on it right next to the director's. We had a brief meeting of the entire cast and crew and received our detailed instructions.

The day was grey, cold and damp. The crash was to occur in heavy rain. This was provided by three large cranes with giant sprinkler heads mounted on top. It rained buckets! I could not believe how realistic it was. To make the woods appear to be burning several artificial, as well as real trees were set ablaze using propane tubes mounted on the trunks. A large propane truck fed the gas to the trees. The resulting fire was very real. In fact, the entire woods seemed to be ablaze. We were told to line up along the retaining wall above the river and await our cue.

When all the actors, cameras, cranes, and support personnel were finally in place the first assistant director gave the command to "Go, Go, Go!" We jumped over the wall and ran slipping and sliding through the blazing trees, down the slope, then to the river's edge. On the way down, I slipped three-stooge like in the mud and fell on my ass, sliding humbly to the bottom of the hill. Retake!

Again, we jumped the wall and raced down the hill. This time I didn't fall. Once at the edge of the river we met Stallone and the other two actors dragging the injured driver through the water. Then we took over. We checked the driver's airway and rapidly applied a cervical collar exactly like we would do in a real crash. Then we dragged him back up the hill, getting drenched by rain the whole time. As we trudged up the hill one of the burning trees fell over with a loud crack, just missing us as we plodded by. No one had bothered to tell us this was going to happen. They wanted us to look surprised. We didn't need to act; it was very, very real!

We did the scene over and over nine times. Each time the assistant director wanted a different camera angle or a slightly different response from one of the actors. After 10 hours of work, we finally got it right. The amazing thing to me was how relaxed, calm, and friendly all of the actors were with each other and with us. We were all soaking wet, cold, and hungry when the day ended. I had forgotten I had ever been sick. My wife was 100% right.

That night we found a great Brazilian restaurant and stuffed ourselves with barbeque and caiparinhas. I hadn't had so much fun in a long time. I called Lynne and probably sounded like I was eight years old. We headed back to the hotel after dinner eagerly anticipating the second day.

When I got to my room, there was a packet under the door. I opened it and found a typewritten document explaining the hazards of the next day's filming. There were to be three helicopters flying together at close range, perhaps flying as low as 30 feet off the ground. Two were to be camera choppers, the third would be the rescue helicopter used as part of the act. The rain-making cranes would still be in place, adding to the hazard of the trees already there. The letter informed me that there would be divers and paramedics in place to rescue me if things went wrong. It further stated that if I wanted to get out of the deal, now was the time to say so. I didn't give any thought to not being there the next morning!

The scene the next day was awesome! Wind, rain, fire, falling trees, helicopters, noise, ambulances, firetrucks, bull horns, rescue personnel, divers, it was wonderful. We rescued the injured driver nine or 10 more times. The assistant director was finally happy and we left town later that night, wired for our next race.

The movie, *Driven,* came out in May. I was invited to the premier held in Los Angeles. I could hardly wait! I arrived at the theater with Joe Heitzler, CART's new CEO, in a big white limousine. We arrived just behind Stallone in his. This was unreal. Gawking people lined both sides of the street. We entered the theater on a long red carpet as driver Paul Tracy entertained the crowd doing doughnuts in the street with his CART car. My excitement level rose dramatically.

The theater was packed. The film began with a gorgeous scene from Long Beach. My heart was racing. This was potentially the biggest thing to ever happen to CART. What a promotion. Our fan base should quadruple, TV ratings should skyrocket. This was just what CART needed!

It was downhill from there. The movie basically sucked! The crash scenes were comical. There were some brief interludes with excellent acting, especially from the old pros, Stallone and Burt Reynolds. The women were beautiful and some of the photography was exceptional. The rest of the movie was disjointed, overplayed and amateurish. The 'big' crash scene was less than 45 seconds long and truly ridiculous. The Safety Team was in the film for a total of maybe three seconds. Three days and a reported 2.4 million dollars were consumed in making that scene. I heard later that the movie eventually made some money. It's all about the money. Oh well, I still had a terrific time and I learned a lot. I'm very thankful Lynne made me go to Montreal.

Chapter 32

DEATH IN DAYTONA

The 2000 season came and went without any serious incidents. Thank goodness, after the horrors of 1999. Hopefully, we were back to only a few minor injuries. Trammell and I planned to spend most of the off-season collaborating with our engineering colleagues in Europe and the United States.

We were working together on a number of different studies primarily focusing on the prevention of head and neck injuries. Delphi, General Motors, Daimler-Chrysler, and Ford were developing collegial relationships with each other, uncharacteristically working together to solve a number of safety-related problems in racing. Additionally, the Air Force and NASA had developed interest in our work. Astronaut protection in the space shuttle and pilot protection for ejection seat incidents are two problems that could potentially benefit from crash investigation in the motorsports arena.

Every organization connected with it seemed to be jumping on the safety bandwagon, except for one. NASCAR, the biggest U.S. sanctioning body of all, remained strangely aloof. True, they had attended the ICMS meetings, but our original expectations concerning their eventual involvement hadn't materialized. It appeared to me that they attended the meetings primarily to keep informed of what the rest of us were doing. They never presented any data of their own. According to one of their risk managers, the prevailing opinion within NASCAR was that if they continued to leave safety issues up to the individual teams and the tracks, then they would not have the liability when things went wrong. Things were soon to go terribly wrong.

On Sunday February 14, 2001, I had just returned home from waterskiing in the late afternoon. Competitive waterskiing is what I do to stay in shape, relaxed and sane. I decided to watch the end of the Daytona 500 while catching up on some reading. I sat down in my favorite chair and turned on the TV.

The early part of the race isn't that exciting. The usual drivers exchange the lead from time to time, pacing themselves for the banzai run at the end. The finish of the Daytona 500 is another story. It is always exciting and a thrill to watch. This year was no exception. I put down my magazine as Dale Earnhardt began his customary charge for the lead. With three laps left to go, he was driving all over the track trying to keep Sterling Marlin and Jimmy Spencer from getting by his team-mate, Michael Waltrip, who was currently leading. Waltrip just happened to be employed by Dale Earnhardt Inc.

On the last lap, as I watched the battle unfolding in front of millions of other people tuned in around the world, Earnhardt inadvertently pinched the apex of Turn 4. He lost control of his car, made a slight correction, then appeared to drive almost straight into the outer retaining wall. The crash didn't look bad. Serves him right I thought to myself. Waltrip went on to win the race.

I flipped off the TV and picked up my magazine. About 30 minutes later the phone rang. It was Jon Potter.

"Well, Earnhardt's dead!"

"What do you mean?" I said. "No way! That crash was nothing, I just watched it."

I truly thought Potter was kidding. He went on to explain that he had just received a phone call from a police buddy of his who was working security near the sight of the crash. Greg Mullis was a state trooper who normally patrolled the area around Homestead, Florida. He was also a big race fan and never missed a chance to work Daytona. He called Potter right after the crash and told him that Earnhardt had died at the scene. He said he bled to death in his car.

I hurriedly turned the television back on just as NASCAR was making the official announcement. Dale Earnhardt *was* dead. I stood there in stunned disbelief, as did the entire racing world. The car wasn't damaged except for the front end. It looked as if the cockpit was completely intact. I remembered a number of similar crashes that drivers walked away from. A well-built racecar, even a stock car, with a proper seat and a well-fitted restraint system should have provided adequate protection for a driver in this type of crash. What happened?

After hanging up with Potter, I immediately called John Melvin. If anyone had the answers it would be him. He couldn't believe it either. I asked him to speculate on the probable cause of death and he said it was most likely a basilar skull fracture. I didn't know that Melvin had been investigating three other recent deaths in NASCAR, all of whom had died from a basilar skull fracture. One of these deaths was Adam Petty, son of racing star, Kyle Petty. His throttle had stuck wide open on the backstretch in New Hampshire. Unable to stop, he plowed head on into the concrete wall. He died instantly of a basilar skull fracture. All of the NASCAR deaths had occurred during right frontal impacts.

A crash of this type in a stock car causes the driver's body to be thrust forward after the impact. As the torso continues to move forward, upward, and to the right, the shoulder belts eventually come into play and stop the body abruptly. Unfortunately, the head with the helmet attached continues to accelerate as it misses the steering wheel. In a stock car, the driver sits almost upright and very close to the steering wheel for leverage. With nothing to stop the head, the loads on the neck soon reach a critical point causing the ligaments to fail and the skull to separate from the spine. The four large arteries that supply blood to the brain are often severed in the process. Death is usually instantaneous, just as it was in the Rodriguez crash at Laguna Seca in 1999. The driver bleeds to death at the scene.

Dr. Hubbard's HANS device was designed specifically to prevent this type of injury. Sadly, only one or two drivers in NASCAR used the device in 2000. Earnhardt was not one to worry much about safety. His seat was reported to be sub-standard, his belts were worn loosely and were found to be poorly anchored, and he still preferred an open-faced helmet. He probably would not have worn the HANS device even if it were given to him. He had survived many spectacular crashes during his career and maintained a fatalistic approach to racing. Lady luck had finally deserted him in Daytona.

A thorough investigation would later show that a HANS would have saved Earnhardt's life. I had made the device mandatory in CART that year and it was being highly recommended for other series. The tests Dr. Gramling did in Germany were indisputable. The HANS worked in every conceivable crash scenario. NASCAR, with four deaths from the same cause, had a major safety problem to deal with.

The entire NASCAR community was in shock after Earnhardt's death. He was the most popular driver in their series. Fans around the country went into mourning. The next day I received a call from another popular driver, Bobby Labonte. He simply asked me:

"What can we do?"

In the weeks and months following the Earnhardt death, NASCAR was unmercifully attacked by the media. Even the non-motorsports media took up the assault. ESPN radio managed to reach me the night of the crash less than five hours after it happened. They wanted me to speculate as to the cause of death. I wasn't about to do that, but I did discuss driver protection in general and what we did in CART.

The CART office, and who knows who else, had given various reporters my contact numbers. Overnight, I had inadvertently become the national spokesperson on what was wrong in NASCAR. As the week progressed, I was interviewed on CNN, CBS, NBC, ABC, ESPN and all of the local TV channels in Miami. I was quoted in newspapers and magazines throughout the country and abroad. The media wanted to know why NASCAR didn't have a safety team. They wanted to know why there was not a traveling medical director. They wanted to know why their cars could not withstand a crash like our cars did. They wanted to know why NASCAR hadn't adopted the HANS device. They wanted to know why they raced back to the start-finish line after a crash. Since CART was the acknowledged leader in the area of safety, I was the logical person to talk to. I responded to very leading questions by discussing only what CART did and why CART did it that way. I was very careful not to condemn NASCAR directly, or to discuss their operations in any way.

NASCAR was not happy with my explanations. Even though I was careful not to condemn it, the public drew its own conclusions. Everything has a positive side, however, and the publicity surrounding my interviews was good for CART. More people throughout the world learned who CART was and that CART was indeed the world's leader in motorsports safety at the time.

The publicity was good for me as well. Requests for talks and interviews increased. A number of prestigious institutions had contacted me to speak, Cambridge University in England being one of them. The events surrounding the Earnhardt crash made me realize how much of a force Dr. Trammell and I had been for safety over our nearly 30 years of chasing racecars. NASCAR, meanwhile, continued to boil.

Bruce Kennedy, the son-in-law of Big Bill France, approached me during CART's Michigan 500 in July, five months after the Earnhardt crash. He walked up to me with both hands in the pockets of the long coat he was wearing in the mid-summer heat. He refused my outstretched hand. He asked me to back off from the media. He told me that if I had any issues with NASCAR just to call him or Bill and they would discuss them with me. I couldn't believe it!

Shortly after the incident with Kennedy, I was summoned by Chip Ganassi, owner of both a NASCAR and a CART team, at our race in Elkhart Lake, Wisconsin. He told me he wished I would back off NASCAR. I joked about being afraid to start my car, but I was really concerned.

I wasn't alone in discussing NASCAR's problems. The *Orlando*

Sentinel wrote a series of articles comparing NASCAR's deaths with the deaths in other series. Reporter and gutsy author, Ed Hinton, wrote a book exposing many of NASCAR's shortcomings. Earnhardt's crash shockingly revealed the lack of attention paid to safety by NASCAR, the most popular form of motorsport in America.

NASCAR's problems didn't just start with Earnhardt. Both Adam Petty, grandson of the great Richard Petty, and Kenny Irwin had died before Earnhardt. The mechanism was the same, a right frontal crash with a basilar skull fracture. The media storm was slow to die down. The internal investigation into the fatal crashes was finally completed nearly six months after the Daytona race. During that investigation, particular attention was paid to Earnhardt's crash. NASCAR held a nationally televised press conference to announce the results of their investigation.

The crash was more violent than it had appeared. The change in velocity upon contact with the wall was estimated to be around 42 mph, a significant crash. They had also discovered a torn seatbelt. The belt had been manufactured by Bill Simpson's company. Simpson had been in business for years and made some of the finest safety equipment available. He was a former race driver himself and innovator of several safety items. The blame for the crash centered on the failed and improperly anchored seatbelt. Simpson was outraged.

Following the broadcast, NASCAR officials announced several rule changes. These would include improved head surround protection in the cockpit and standardized seatbelt orientation. Crash recorders were added to their cars. A HANS device or something similar to support the head and neck was mandated. NASCAR would establish a regionally based physician and nurse program and open a research and development center in North Carolina. All of these changes were very positive and will ultimately improve the safety of stock car racing. I am convinced that pressure from the media was the prime reason for NASCAR's accelerated response to the recent string of fatalities.

I have never disliked NASCAR and actually enjoy watching many of its events. Racing on the high banks of Daytona, Talladega or the tough track at Dover, is hard to beat. NASCAR had simply lagged behind the other major leagues of auto racing when it came to safety initiatives. Now, as a result of the Earnhardt tragedy, the people there are attacking safety in a big way. A large and active delegation from NASCAR now attends the annual ICMS meetings. Dr. Melvin has been retained by NASCAR as a safety consultant and is working diligently to improve drivers' cockpit protection. I still don't think they like me very much, but the end result of their sudden interest in safety will benefit everyone in racing. They have the resources to make major contributions. All of us in the sport eagerly await the results of their efforts.

Chapter 33

CART SCREWS UP BIG TIME

C ART had major problems of its own in 2001. In April, we traveled to Texas Motor Speedway for our first race at that facility. The track is near Fort Worth and is a very high-banked 1.5-mile oval. The IRL had some great races there and CART's leadership felt that they could put on an even better show. Our cars would be much faster, therefore more exciting. At least that was the theory. To test the facility, CART sent Team Rahal in the middle of the winter to check it out. It was very cold during the test, and driver Kenny Brack wasn't too excited about going fast. After only a few laps, Brack pronounced the track safe. His top speed was reportedly around 206 mph.

Wally Dallenbach had visited the track earlier in the year with technical boss Kirk Russell. They drove around the speedway in a rental car and didn't like what they saw. Both of them went on record against an event at Texas Motor Speedway. They felt that the track was very dangerous because of the high anticipated speeds and the sharp increase in the angle of banking after coming off the relatively flat straightaways. I didn't visit the track personally, but I talked to several of the drivers who told me they thought it was too dangerous. Sadly, Dallenbach, Russell, I and practically every other CART official were overruled by our latest CEO, former CART champion and Indy 500 winner, Bobby Rahal. I think Rahal was the 14th CEO in CART's brief history.

It appeared that Rahal had his own agenda. It was his driver who participated in the winter test and many questioned the test's validity. In spite of all the negatives, we headed for Texas.

I left Miami for Dallas with great trepidation. I had recently talked to Dallenbach and he reinforced the fact that we had no business racing at Texas Motor Speedway. After landing in Dallas, I drove the 40 or so miles to the track and remarked to my wife how wide open the area still seemed to be. It wasn't hard to imagine a big cattle drive as they were portrayed in so many movies. After an hour or so of flat, monotonous plain the grandstands loomed in the distance.

The track was an awesome facility, a great place to showcase the NASCAR Nextel Cup Series but not us. During Friday's practice session our cars hit a staggering 232 mph *average* speed. It seemed that the engineers had figured out a lot over the winter. The drivers were lapping the 24 degree banking in less than 20 seconds. Trammell and I crossed our fingers.

Early in the Friday practice period a very fast Cristiano da Matta crashed in the second turn. Thankfully, he wasn't injured, but his car was totaled. No explanation was given for the crash. Later in the afternoon, Mauricio Gugelmin crashed hard exiting the same turn. He lost control in almost the exact same spot as da Matta. Gugelmin's crash was far more severe.

Following what appeared to be a normal racing line, he suddenly lost control and crashed nose-first into the outside retaining wall. The crash recorder registered 66 G. This is a big front-end crash! The impact nearly flattened his headrest and caused his right foot to wedge between the brake pedal and the throttle. The throttle stuck wide open as a consequence. The wrecked car continued to accelerate. Gugelmin was just a passenger as his car hurtled down the backstretch at full throttle. It hit the wall again in the third turn after spinning 180 degrees. This second impact registered 113 G. His headrest was now totally used up.

Remarkably, Mauricio was still conscious. His car still hadn't stopped after the second impact and was headed for a third impact with its nosecone totally removed. At this juncture, his feet were completely exposed. He was headed directly toward Dr. Trammell in Safety 2. If he hit a third time he would never walk again. Luckily, the car came to a stop a short distance in front of Safety 2. When the Safety Team arrived, Gugelmin was awake and appeared to be uninjured. A double impact of this magnitude would have been fatal just a few years earlier. Thankfully, he was wearing his HANS device. Without it he would likely have been killed.

The Safety Team was able to extricate him without difficulty. Usually very analytical, Guglemin was dumbfounded as to why he crashed. He was convinced something had broken in the car. He kept staring toward the second turn, perplexed.

The ambulance brought him to the medical unit for his compulsory examination. There, Dr. Trammell and I inspected his HANS device and found that it was badly fractured. We had not seen that before. Without it, those fractures would have been in his neck. The scary thing about the crash was that not only Gugelmin but no one else had an explanation for it. His crew could find nothing that had broken in the car. The observers reported a normal racing line before his sudden loss of control. Telemetry had not registered any malfunctions in any of the car's systems. The cause remained a mystery.

Trammell and I went back and talked to da Matta again. He didn't have any idea as to the cause of his crash either, nor did his crew. The situation was really troubling. Usually, there is a satisfactory explanation for most crashes. Nothing had broken on either car and the drivers were clueless. Terry and I were very concerned and discussed the incidents at dinner that evening. Dallenbach was troubled as well and told us to be ready because it was going to be a busy weekend!

Saturday morning dawned crystal clear and very comfortable for April in Texas. During the morning practice session Paul Tracy reached a blistering average speed of 236 mph. All but two of the cars were over the 230 mph barrier. Amazingly, no one crashed. Nevertheless, we were still on high alert as the speeds continued to climb. I had a sickening feeling of impending doom. With the ability to draft, the race speeds would be even faster. Two cars

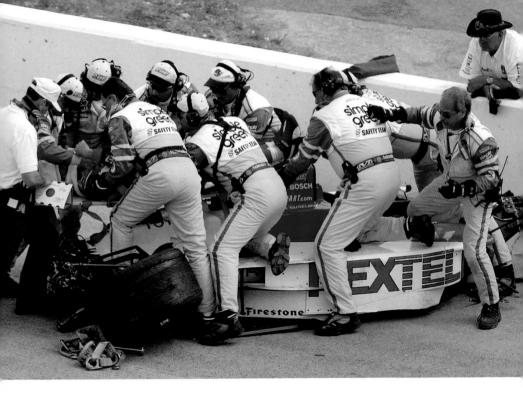

ABOVE *The Safety Team extricating driver Mauricio Gugelmin following his huge accident at Texas Motor Speedway in 2001. The potentially fatal crash was caused by the combination of both high vertical and lateral G.* (Getty Images)

BELOW *Explaining to drivers the high G-loads experienced by Paul Tracy on his record-breaking lap of over 236 mph at Texas World Speedway.* (Motorsport Images)

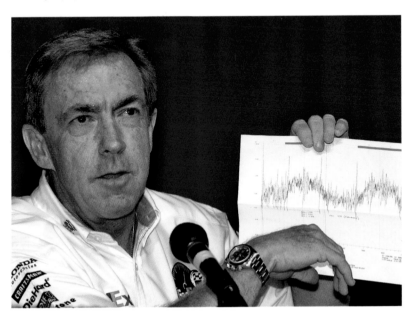

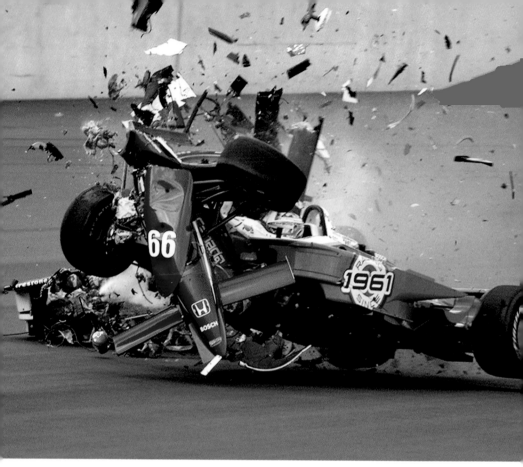

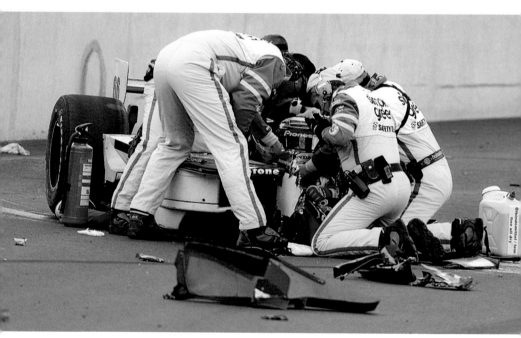

OPPOSITE TOP *The terrible moment of impact as Alex Tagliani spears Alex Zanardi's Reynard at the Lausitzring Eurospeedway in 2001.* (Getty Images)

OPPOSITE BOTTOM *The Safety Team works feverishly to save Zanardi.* (Getty Images)

RIGHT *Zanardi pays a surprise visit to Toronto less than a year after losing both legs in the German Memorial race.* (Dan R. Boyd)

BELOW *Two years after the accident Zanardi completes the symbolic final 13 laps of his truncated race at Lausitzring, putting to bed his horrible ordeal.* (Motorsport Images)

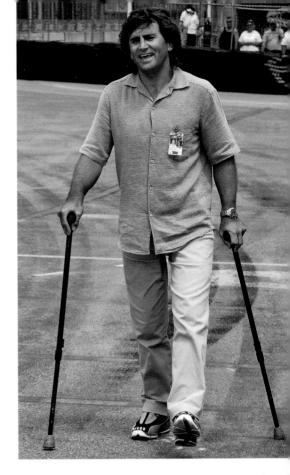

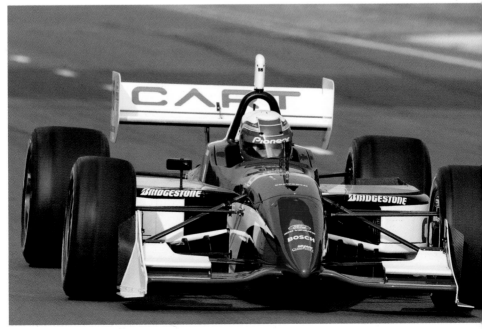

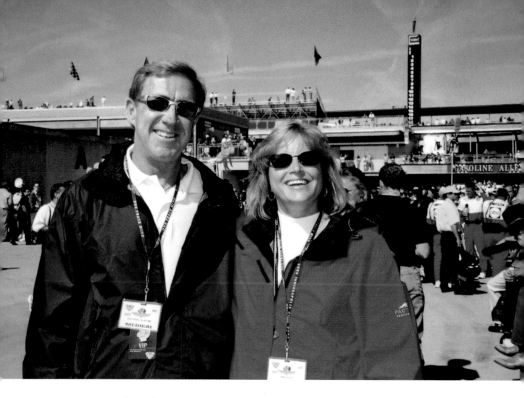

ABOVE *The author and his wife, Lynne, at Indy on race morning.* (Author)

BELOW *The crash at Daytona in February 2001 that took stock car legend Dale Earnhardt's life.* (Motorsport Images)

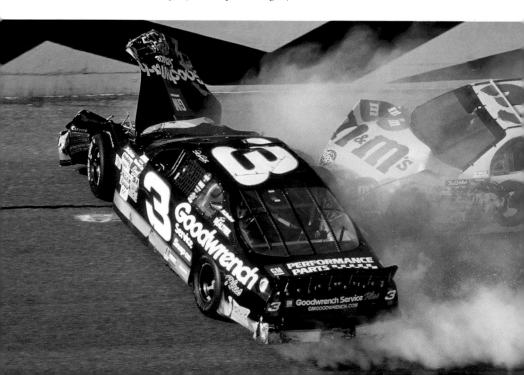

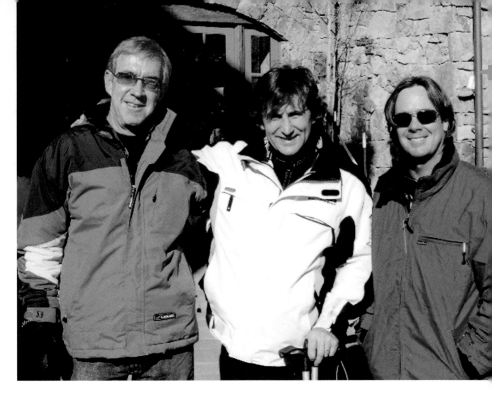

ABOVE *The author hooks up with Jimmy Vasser and Alex Zanardi at Beaver Creek, Colorado, for some off-season skiing.* (Author)

BELOW LEFT *Wally Dallenbach sporting his famous hat, in command on the CART circuit.* (Dan R. Boyd)

BELOW RIGHT *The legendary A.J. Foyt – what more needs to be said?* (Dan R. Boyd)

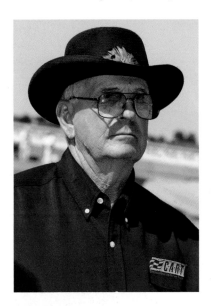

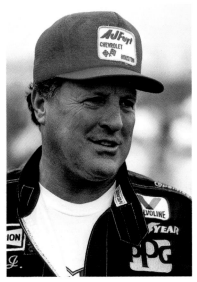

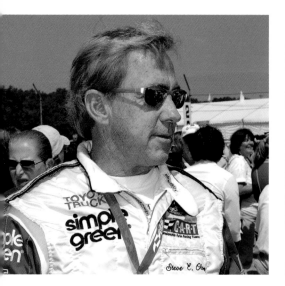

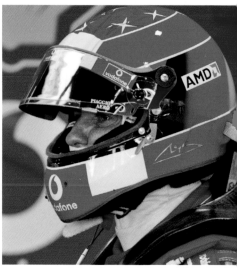

ABOVE LEFT *The author in anticipation of a good day.* (Dan R. Boyd)

ABOVE RIGHT *Multiple Formula One champion Michael Schumacher wears the life-saving HANS device.* (Motorsport Images)

BELOW *Professor Sid Watkins, flanked by Dr. Hugh Scully and the author at the Prof's home in Scotland for Hogmanay 2004.* (Author)

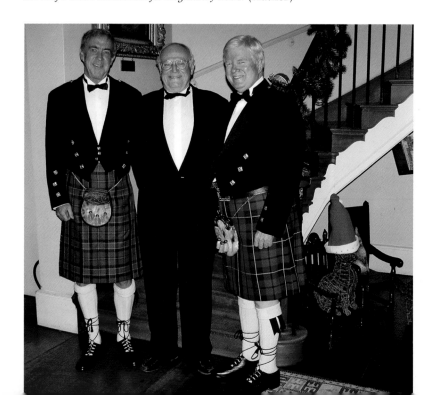

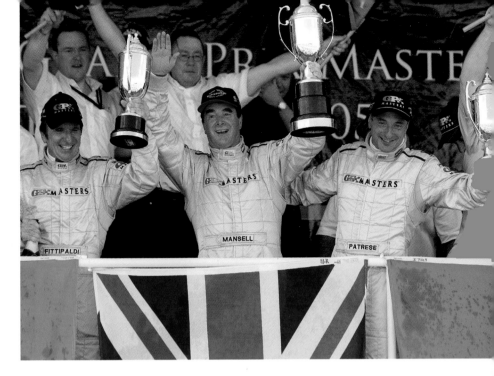

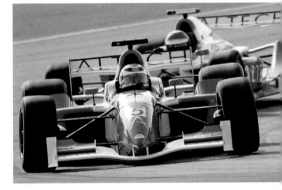

ABOVE *Like children at Christmas. The victorious Nigel Mansell, flanked by fellow podium finishers Emerson Fittipaldi (left) and Riccardo Patrese, celebrate at Kyalami in 2005 after proving in the Grand Prix Masters race they still have what it takes.* (Motorsport Images)

MIDDLE *Nigel Mansell on his way to winning the closely contested Grand Prix Masters race in Qatar in 2006, perhaps the hottest race ever recorded!* (Motorsport Images)

RIGHT *The author with Roger Penske at the Homestead, Florida IRL race in March 2006, two months before 'The Captain' would steer his team to its 14th Indy 500 victory.* (Author)

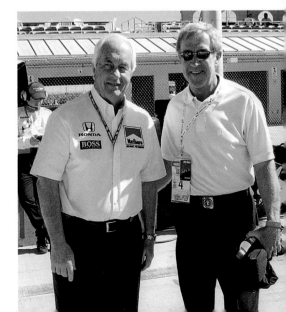

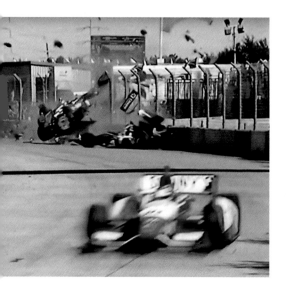
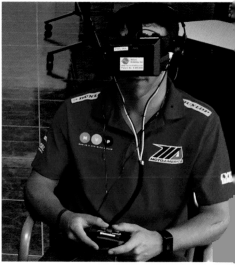

ABOVE LEFT *Dario Franchitti, airborne and spinning violently at Houston in 2013. With no significant impact with the barrier, his concussion was due to the rapid rotation of his head.* (YouTube)

ABOVE RIGHT *A subject being tested for concussion. The device resembles a bad pair of binoculars, but measures a substantial amount of data.* (Author)

BELOW *Will Power ready to race in 2018, head nestled into the head surround to limit rotation in the event of a crash.* (Author)

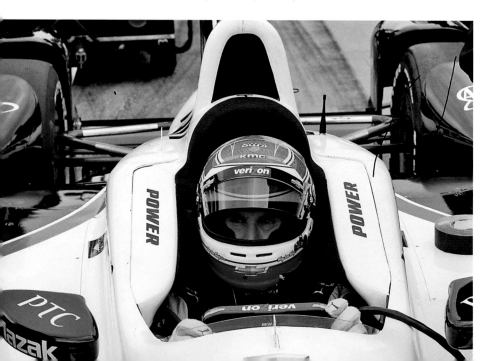

running nose-to-tail with each other creates a vacuum between them that effectively gives each car more horsepower.

About halfway through the morning practice, Canadian driver Patrick Carpentier visited the medical unit. Trammell had fixed his wrist fracture a few weeks before and wanted me to check it after he had driven a few hot laps. While I was examining his wrist, the driver told me something very curious. He said that when he climbed out of his racecar he had to sit down immediately on the pit wall for a few seconds to avoid falling over. He was very concerned because he had never experienced a feeling like that before.

Not sure what was going on, I told him that it was probably his inner ear acting up, the result of having to fly so often. I examined his ears and throat and they looked fine. I told him to be careful and to let me know if the feeling returned. I had seen inner ear problems with drivers in the past and they occasionally required treatment.

Kathi Lauterbach, the perky, beautiful and very smart PR director for Newman-Haas Racing, bounded into the unit shortly after I had released Carpentier. She looked very concerned and told me she had just overheard an alarming conversation between Brazilian drivers Helio Castroneves and Tony Kanaan; two of the fastest. They were on different teams, but still remained good friends from their earlier days racing karts in Brazil. They were complaining to each other about feeling dizzy and sick to their stomachs. Kathi heard them say that they felt as if they were spinning around while they were actually in the car at speed. They couldn't tell for sure if they were right side up!

What they were describing sounded like vertigo, often a symptom of an inner ear problem. Vertigo, unlike dizziness, is usually due to some significant problem like an inner ear infection or even a brain tumor. I doubted that three different drivers would be having inner ear problems at the same time, especially veteran drivers who were used to the lifestyle and the high speeds. I remembered reading an article discussing G-loads on fighter pilots and the thought struck me that we might be dealing with a similar experience. Bad deal!

I thanked Kathi and hurriedly left the unit looking for Paul Tracy's team manager. I might as well look at the telemetry data on the fastest driver. I found Tracy's manager in the team's transporter and asked him if I could see the in-car data sheet, usually highly proprietary information. I was hoping that it would show me the G-loads experienced by the driver. Tracy's manager showed me the graph. I was shocked to find that Paul was experiencing more than 3.5 vertical G. Race drivers normally don't experience much in the way of vertical G at all. Coupled with the high vertical G the graph showed lateral G of 5.5, sustained in the fastest part of the race track! We had seen lateral G of this magnitude before on some of our tighter road courses, but never coupled with increased vertical G. I was convinced we were having a problem with excessive G loading due to the high speeds and the geometry of this particular race track.

This combination of G forces is very dangerous. We were headed for a major catastrophe. Needing back up, I sought out aviation expert Dr. Richard Jennings, formerly the flight director for NASA and the only G-force expert I knew. I met him years earlier through Dr. Bock at the Speedway in Indianapolis. He now lived in the Houston area only a few hours from the Texas track. He had written his doctoral thesis on the gravitational effects of flying supersonic jets. I needed to find Jennings quickly.

I hurriedly paged him, left a message for him at work, and called his home. I waited anxiously. No luck. No return call. More than an hour elapsed. Still no word! The next practice session was due to start in less than an hour. I began to panic.

I paged Dr. Jennings a second time, growing more anxious by the minute. About to give up, I suddenly felt a gentle hand on my right shoulder. I looked up and caught my breath. He was standing there with that big smile of his spread from ear to ear. He had decided to drive up from Houston on a whim. It was a miracle!

"Boy, I'm sure glad to see you!" I yelled.

I quickly showed him the data and he remarked very calmly: "You're in big trouble!"

"Shit!" I think I said.

I immediately called for Wally Dallenbach and Joe Heitzler. Formerly a sales and marketing guy for CBS, Heitzler took on the tenuous position of CEO after Rahal quit in December. When Heitzler and Dallenbach arrived, I showed them the data and gave them my opinion. Jennings backed me up. Dallenbach cancelled the next session.

Jennings then gave me a crash course on G forces and the human body. He informed me that amusement parks don't build rollercoasters to exceed 3.5 vertical G because they want to thrill the customers not make them sick. Pilots in the military have to don their G suits if they plan to exceed 4 G in their fighter jets. No one had ever studied the effects of combining high vertical G with high lateral G, according to Jennings. The combination of G forces shown on Tracy's data sheet had never happened before. At least it had never been recorded anywhere in the scientific literature. We were entering uncharted territory!

Heitzler called an emergency drivers' meeting. No one outside of Dallenbach, Heitzler, Jennings or me had any clue what was happening. I told Trammell the news as soon as he came in from the track. He and the other safety guys had been sitting on station for over an hour waiting for word from the Chief Steward. They had no idea what was going on. Terry was in disbelief.

The drivers were hurriedly assembled in their meeting room and I was given the floor following a few brief remarks from Heitzler. I asked if any of them had experienced any dizziness, vertigo, lost awareness, visual disturbances, nausea, vomiting or any other unusual symptoms. To the amazement of everyone in the room, 18 of the 20 drivers had suffered some or all of these symptoms. One admitted to losing complete awareness from the time he entered the second turn until the time he exited the third turn during his fastest lap. He had wisely pulled into his pit, scared! He told me after the meeting that he thought he was having a stroke. What he had experienced is what pilots call G-loc. It is a momentary loss of consciousness as a result of decreased blood flow to the brain caused by excessive G.

Drivers, being the macho individuals that they are, usually won't admit to any frailties. The only way to get them to admit to any kind of disability is to get them together as a group. Once one of them opens up, the rest will usually follow. The two drivers who had not experienced any symptoms had driven less than four consecutive laps. It became apparent that, depending on how fast they went, all of them would become symptomatic after eight to 10 laps. We were in *big* trouble!

CART did not want to cancel the race under any circumstances. Everything was in place, tickets had been sold, and live TV was scheduled. We would look really foolish in the eyes of the media, the fans, and the promoter. A cancellation would cost CART a ton of money. The obvious question being asked was how could the IRL race there so successfully? The answer is scientific. G force is a function of the square of the velocity, in other words there is a geometric progression in the G forces as the velocity increases. The IRL had never gone over 225 mph, and our increase of 11 mph caused a huge rise in the level of G. Jennings and I determined from looking at the speed charts that an average speed of less than 229 mph was probably safe. It was not until a driver exceeded 229 mph that trouble developed. Tolerance to increasing G loads varies in individuals and some of the drivers took several laps to develop symptoms.

With the scientific information in hand, a second meeting was called that included the owners, the track's management, the tire representatives and representatives from each of the engine manufacturers, Honda, Toyota and Ford. Heitzler called the meeting to order at 2:00 in the afternoon. It lasted until 11:30 that night! During those nine and a half hours every conceivable method to slow the cars down was discussed. Any changes made to the engines would result in blown units and the associated risk of serious accidents. There was nothing that could be done to the tires at that late date. A change in track configuration would require road course parts being exchanged on the cars so they could turn right and those parts were back at the respective race shops. CART was stuck!

It canceled the race the next morning. For the first time in history a race was canceled for medical reasons. It is a tribute to Heitzler that he had the guts to back up his medical director. After the announcement Roger Penske glared at me in disgust. Not believing the science, he had his drivers dress for the race anyway.

Heitzler and I were immediately surrounded by the media. Headlines the next day would read; "Daring Doctor Cancels Race." Eddie Gossage, the track's operating officer, was furious. Highly skeptical, he instantly threatened CART with a lawsuit. It was a grim day for all concerned. The teams reluctantly packed up to go home. Several thousand fans had already arrived for the race and were also told to go home. CART would eventually refund their money, but there were an awful lot of hard feelings. The next morning the decision made national news. I received phone calls from all over the country. Even the Pentagon called. An admiral was very interested in our data and wanted to know if we would be willing to share it with the Navy. Also interested was Dr. Knox at Wright-Patterson AFB and Jennings said that he had talked to a bigwig in NASA, and they were also intrigued.

I returned the call to the Pentagon as soon as I returned to Miami. The admiral informed me that the Navy had just completed an experiment looking at the effects of combined vertical and lateral G on pilots. They were studying these combined G-load effects because of jets they had on the drawing board. Called agile aircraft, these jets would be able to turn without banking due to the ability of variably directing their engine nozzles during flight allowing them to achieve level flight in all attitudes. Turning suddenly without banking in a supersonic aircraft would create some very high lateral G. Conventional aircraft don't experience high lateral G because pilots are able to bank the plane when they turn. No one knew if humans would be physically able to fly these newly designed aircraft if and when they were ever built. Tests were conducted in the Navy and Air Force to determine if these planes could be flown at all.

One test performed by the Navy subjected a number of pilots to a gimbaled centrifuge where both vertical and lateral G could be produced. Using only 1.5 lateral G coupled with modest vertical G, they were startled by the results. Within a very short time all of the pilots in the study developed temporary blindness in their inside eye. Had we raced in Texas all of our drivers would have been blind in their left eye within one or two laps! The result would be no depth perception. Suicide at 230 mph!

The Navy findings were released soon after our Texas debacle. Dr. Jennings presented CART's experience to his friends in NASA as well as at the annual Aerospace Medical Association meeting. All of the experts agreed that CART made the correct and only decision it could. We likely saved lives, but the cancellation of the race eventually cost CART over three million dollars! From now on, sanctioning bodies would have to consider anticipated G forces when designing and building race tracks.

The mystery of the two practice crashes was now solved. Excessive G loads not only affect blood flow to the eye and brain, they also affect the inner ear. When this occurs, the ear sends the wrong message to the brain regarding spatial orientation. In both cases, the drivers' brains were being told by their ears that they were losing control of their cars. In reality, they were under perfect control. This false information caused them to correct a non-existent slip of the rear end, resulting in a loss of control. The outcome for each driver was a big crash! The sensation both drivers felt was similar to the feeling we all felt as a child when we rode the playground merry-go-round. As soon as you jumped off, even though you were walking a straight line, you felt as if you were spinning out of control. CART was now spinning out of control.

It had to live with the Texas decision the entire season of 2001. Even though knowledgeable people knew the right decision had been made, CART could not escape the fact that it had gone to Texas in the first place. The CART leadership had bumbled again. Another series sponsor was irked. Fed-Ex, the primary sponsor, announced they were leaving at the end of the year as had PPG, Cadillac, GMC, Hilton Hotels, and others before them. CART's TV contract was in a shambles and there was generalized disagreement on the direction CART should take in the future. Remarkably, CART had no long-range plan in place. Its direction seemed to change on a daily basis.

Rumors were rampant about team defections to the IRL. The biggest rumor had Roger Penske jumping ship in 2002, likely taking Toyota's engine program with him. It appeared that CART's luster of the early and mid-90s was fading fast. Crowds on the oval tracks had decreased steadily since 1997. Before that, CART regularly outdrew NASCAR. Teams were now having more and more difficulty obtaining sponsorships as companies flocked to NASCAR's Winston Cup series. NASCAR was growing exponentially while CART had rapidly begun to fade.

CART had never grasped the importance of catering to the media. They often treated the media as rabble, unfit for serious consideration. As a result, the motorsports press enjoyed taking pot shots at CART whenever the chance arose, and it arose often. Internally, morale among the officials was at an all-time low. It was difficult for the rank and file to comprehend how CART could have survived through so many less-than-competent CEOs, all of whom left the company with bulging pockets. CART, it seemed, was a large cash cow that only a select few were able to milk. On top of that, the nation's economy was beginning to falter and the CART Board was in turmoil following a number of key resignations. Chip Ganassi and Roger Penske both resigned from the CART Board during the 2001 season. Trammell and I continued to do our jobs naively hoping that somehow everything would eventually work out for the best.

Chapter 34

HEAD INJURY AND RETURN
TO COMPETITION

The mood in the paddock continued to deteriorate throughout the 2001 season. Everyone, the suppliers, the sponsors, the owners, the fans and the drivers were increasingly concerned about the future of CART. Terry and I, in spite of the gloom and doom, continued to pursue the science of injury cause and effect. During this period of frustration with CART, the media brought to the surface a problem within the National Football League that had important consequences for many sports. Repeated minor head injury has been a smoldering issue within all contact sports for years. The retirements of Steve Young and Troy Aikman brought the problem into the public's eye. For several years, I had worried about the possible effects of drivers having too many concussions. At one point, several years ago, I had entertained the idea of having one of our drivers tested to determine if he had a balance and perception problem related to too many minor head injuries during his career. I had gone so far as to make arrangements with the military to test him in a centrifuge. The driver in question was crashing repeatedly for no apparent cause. Fortunately, he retired of his own volition just before I received clearance to do the test.

Until 2001, we had no sure way to evaluate an athlete following a minor head injury. The consensus for return to competition was based on studies done by Dr. Robert Cantu, the guru of concussion in sports. Concussions were divided into grades based primarily on duration of lost consciousness. Return to competition was based on a safe guess rather than real data. Driving for CART back in the mid-90s, Robby Gordon crashed at the Michigan speedway on

Friday afternoon and was unconscious for less than three minutes. He woke up completely, and was fine the next day. He probably could have raced on Sunday but the guidelines said he had to wait out an entire week. Gordon was mad, but there was nothing else I could do. On several occasions, athletes were allowed to return to a sport too soon simply because they wanted to play and some unqualified physician said it was OK. NASCAR, until very recently, would accept a note from any physician attesting to a driver being able to compete safely after a period of lost consciousness. Dale Earnhardt Jr. admitted to the press that he probably should not have been driving after a bad crash in 2004.

Researchers at the University of Pittsburgh have been studying minor head injury as an issue for some time. One of the leading investigators is a doctor by the name of Mark Lovell who, along with neurosurgeon Joe Maroon, designed a revolutionary computer-based neuropsychological test called ImPACT. This new test can be administered via a laptop computer in the field within minutes of a blow to the head. The results can then be compared to a baseline study obtained at the beginning of the season. If an athlete deviated too far from his baseline, he was determined to have had a concussion and was kept out of play. He was not allowed to return to competition until a repeat test closely matched his baseline. Sometimes it is safe to return to competition within 48 hours after a minor concussion, other times the ImPACT score would not approach baseline for several weeks.

Dr. Lovell contacted me during the winter of 2001–2002 and asked if I would be interested in the ImPACT program for CART. No one knows how many drivers in the past had continued racing long after they should have retired, or how many were injured, or may have injured someone else after returning too soon. Dr. Lovell's research also showed that you didn't need to be knocked out to have had a significant injury to the brain. This was new information at the time. Always before, the gold standard for diagnosing a concussion was loss of consciousness. I looked forward to having a test that could precisely identify when a driver had suffered an injury to the brain and when a driver could resume his career.

CART was the first motorsports organization to adopt the ImPACT program, setting the industry standard of care once again. It is hoped that with ImPACT drivers in the future will not risk early dementia, loss of employment, personality changes or any of the other consequences of repeated mild traumatic brain injury.

Terry and I continued to strengthen our relationship with Professor Watkins. One of the most interesting characters you would ever like to meet, he developed similar programs in Europe and spearheaded, along with Dr. Scully, the drive to unite both sides of the Atlantic in the mutual pursuit of racing safety. He had invited both of us to attend the inaugural United States Grand Prix held at the Speedway in Indianapolis in 2000. To my surprise, he had arranged for me to spend the day in the hallowed Ferrari garage and pit area. I thought CART was hi-tech. Wrong! Formula One, and Ferrari especially, were light years ahead of anything I had ever seen in CART. Using satellite signals the Ferrari engineers were able to make adjustments to the car all the way from Italy. Few words were spoken within the Ferrari garage. The crew members all knew their jobs and went about their work without needing to say anything. The two drivers behaved like robots coming out of their separate dressing rooms and getting into their respective cars. No words were spoken as Michael Schumacher garnered his zillionth pole position.

While I was enjoying myself in the Ferrari garage, Terry was stuck in the infield hospital. The mistake he made was agreeing to be on Dr. Bock's medical staff for the Grand Prix. He had been issued a medical pass, not a cherished paddock pass from the exalted Bernie Eccelestone. Unlike the CART races, the medical staff for a Formula One event does not enjoy full access to the track and grounds. The pass Terry was given allowed him to visit the infield hospital and surrounding compound only. That first year he didn't get to see anything but white sheets, the TV monitor and Dr. Bock's nurses.

We did get to meet formally with Professor Watkins and Dr. Gary Hartstein, the Belgian-based American anesthesiologist who replaced Watkins in 2005. We enjoyed dinner and formed an alliance to share research interests and crash data. This was a major step in international motorsports diplomacy. Before, Formula One and American racing had always remained a good arm's length from each other. Throughout the winter of 2001 Trammell and I kept in close contact with Watkins, Hartstein and the other FIA stalwarts. Returning to Indy for the Formula One race in 2001, we agreed to look into the feasibility of sharing a common database with the FIA.

Trammell had been studying the HANS device since its introduction. He had actually written several prescriptions for it to be used by several sprint and midget car drivers who had suffered otherwise career-ending neck injuries. Formula One was ready to introduce the HANS into their series and needed Dr. Trammell's input. The FIA flew him to Brazil to meet with the drivers. He explained the value of the HANS to the likes of Michael Schumacher, enjoyed Brazil, and saw the Grand Prix as a VIP. I felt he was adequately compensated for his ordeal the year before at Indy.

Chapter 35

CART AUGERS IN

It looked like Team Penske would win the CART championship for the umpteenth time in 2001. The 26th annual Colorado 500 had come and gone and I missed out again. Due to our expanded race schedule, and my heavy commitment to the University, I began to doubt if I would ever get my 10th ride in. I had skied well in the National Water Ski tournament in Bakersfield, California in August, finishing 26th in the Men's V division. My children were all doing well and the grandchildren were into everything. Like most Americans, I really had nothing big to complain about. It was late summer already. Where had the year gone?

On Labor Day weekend, Terry and I had been enjoying Vancouver, B.C. The race had just ended with no serious crashes. We decided to have dinner that evening at the great Italian place we could never remember the name of. We soon found ourselves sipping vodka and discussing the state of affairs in CART. We had nothing else to do, the night was young, and we weren't scheduled to fly out until dawn the next morning.

The rumors about Roger Penske had grown louder. He had recently dumped all of his CART stock and had resigned from the CART Board of Directors. Some of the CART regulars thought Penske had finally had enough of Pat Patrick and Carl Haas, not the easiest businessmen to get the best of. Most of us thought he was simply preparing to defect to the IRL.

Whether he willed it or not, if Penske did defect to the IRL, CART would most likely die a slow and agonizing death. Penske had won the Indy 500 that May for the 11th time. He won it with the brash young Brazilian, Helio Castroneves. It was the second year in a row for a CART driver to win the IRL's big event. Juan Pablo Montoya, the 1999 CART champion, won in 2000 driving for owner Chip Ganassi. The strength of CART was an embarrassment for the fledgling IRL.

Roger Penske loved Indy. His 11 wins there were more than any other owner in the history of the sport. Many felt that he could not resist the lure of the Indianapolis Motor Speedway. Almost all race fans wanted the two series to get back together as one strong American open-wheeled championship. Nothing on the horizon even hinted about any kind of successful union.

As Terry and I pondered his next move, we couldn't help but think if Penske goes, who will follow? Penske was fairly vocal in his desire to have only one U.S. open-wheeled series. For him, that would have to include the Indy 500. He would have to join the IRL if he was to save Indy, now in jeopardy because of the split with CART. TV ratings were dropping annually and for the first time anyone could remember tickets were not hard to come by for the famous race. For the IRL to win the battle, CART would have to go away or at least become a virtual motorsport non-entity. But how could he destroy CART?

To kill CART we surmised, all Penske needed to do was convince his engine company to leave the series with him. Once Toyota left, Honda would likely follow. Rumors had it that the only reason Honda was in racing at all was to beat its arch rival Toyota. Then, like the proverbial house of cards, CART would fall.

The engine companies had grown extremely powerful in CART over the previous decade, providing a substantial amount of the team's operating budgets. In fact, those two engine suppliers were reported to account for nearly 60% of the CART team's total support. Losing Toyota and Honda would eliminate all but a few of CART's strongest teams. It would mean that many of the CART teams would have to defect if they were to stay solvent. This is indeed what happened.

Toyota announced its defection in concert with Penske. Honda soon followed, taking Michael Andretti and Team Green with them. Other defectors would include Chip Ganassi Racing, Morris Nunn Racing, and one car each from both Team Rahal and Fernandez Racing. Patrick Racing would eventually leave as well. If CART did fold, anyone wishing to race Indycars would have to be in the IRL. By leaving CART, Penske had started a chain reaction that seemed likely to force all open-wheeled racers into the IRL, therefore saving the Indy 500 from further deterioration and hopefully allowing open-wheeled racing to regain the stature it had lost during the split.

As the night wore on, Terry and I were getting more and more depressed. No one, it seemed, could deal with CART's largely incompetent infrastructure. As a result of CART's colossal ineptness, new sponsors were not knocking the doors down. CART, it seemed, had no friends. Mainstream media gave little notice to the series, the TV package had to be purchased, and the fan base was diminishing with the exception of the Mexican and Canadian markets.

NASCAR, who could have been a great partner with CART, was angrily aligning itself with the IRL. Through its International Speedway Corporation, NASCAR now owned and operated several race tracks around the country. In 2000, CART raced at many of them, including tracks in Michigan, California, Florida, and Pennsylvania. CART, because of dwindling oval track crowds, rather stupidly dropped the ISC tracks from the schedule. This infuriated NASCAR. It was like a little dog lifting his leg on the big elephant. CART placed itself in great jeopardy when it allowed the IRL and NASCAR to get into bed with each other.

To add fuel to the fire, it was no secret to anyone that Toyota wanted desperately to get on the NASCAR bandwagon. This was likely one of the cards Penske played to get Toyota to desert CART with him in the first place. Penske had a lot of influence in NASCAR and could expedite Toyota's participation.

It all seemed so logical. Terry and I were now in deep despair. If CART folded we were in a major quandary. NASCAR didn't like us and the IRL didn't need us. We realized that we might have to explore other options if and when CART ceased to exist. We were thankful for the relationship we had developed with the FIA. They were the governing body of motorsports worldwide and there were rumors of a new FIA Institute for Motorsports Safety in the works.

Other changes were rumored in CART. Joe Heitzler was said to be on the chopping block. The Texas fiasco, although not his fault, coupled with a bad TV deal, were among the reasons given. The man in line to replace Heitzler was rumored to be expatriate Englishman Christopher Pook, the founder of the very successful Long Beach Grand Prix. Long Beach was the only known street venue to ever make a substantial profit. Pook was a well-respected member of the motorsports community. He and Bernie Ecclestone had worked together in Formula One in the distant past, so he was still well connected.

Gaining prominence with a longshoreman's tough guy attitude, Pook persisted, coerced and pleaded with the city of Long Beach to establish his Grand Prix way back in 1976, after staging a Formula 5000 race there in 1975. He was known to speak his mind, occasionally without due regard for the consequences. Most of us thought he was the only man who could save CART, if CART was indeed salvageable. Trammell and I hoped that Pook favored a strong medical and safety program, and that he would continue to support all of our research efforts. As Terry said:

"We invented the car; we certainly didn't want to become the trailer."

Our medical delivery system, our seats, our head-surround, our push for the HANS device, our ear accelerometers, our data collection, and our scientific publications had all led the way in motorsports safety. Bits and pieces of the work we had done together were now used in Formula One, the IRL, and NASCAR, not to mention many other series including the unlimited hydroplanes, drag racers, and various sportscar organizations. NASCAR was slowly adopting the seating principles developed in CART and CART's cockpit protection devices, although it did not want to admit it. Now almost everyone uses the HANS device. Our system for on-track rescue is widely imitated and often written about. Every other safety system in motorsports is compared to ours. With Lon Bromley, we had become the gold standard! We were determined to maintain our position as the world leader. We thought we could only do this if CART survived.

From its inception CART was often plagued with greedy, selfish and arrogant owners who seemed to push their own agendas regardless of the consequences. Individual owners controlled parts, engines or whole cars. Because these owners collectively made up the board of directors, nothing sustaining, with the exception of the Safety Team, was ever accomplished. Unlike NASCAR, CART never marketed the drivers as heroes and athletes. A few drivers, such as Emerson Fittipaldi and Mario Andretti, the Unsers, Foyt, and Rutherford were able to successfully market themselves, but they had virtually no help from CART. Most of the CART drivers could walk around any large city totally unrecognized. Unbelievably, CART has no written history of its own. Employees come and go with little or no recognition of ever having been there.

CART once hired a young attractive marketing person whose first race was at the California Speedway. As part of her orientation, she was offered a pace car ride with Wally Dallenbach, famous throughout the world of motor racing. As Dallenbach entered the first turn she turned to him and said casually:

"Gee Wally; did you ever think you might want to drive a racecar?"

CART is 25 years old! Wally's been there since day one. Ask people on the street what CART stands for and 99 out of 100 won't have a clue. Egos and jealousies within the organization continued to hamper sponsorship efforts as well as alienate important players outside of CART's inner circle. At times CART, as the company, would be in direct competition with its own teams for sponsorship. CART was quickly running out of gas.

Meanwhile, the IRL was doggedly hanging in there. Largely financed by Tony George, it had managed to stay in business.

Embarrassed by its dismal showing at the Indianapolis 500 in 2000 and 2001, it was desperate to beat CART no matter what the cost. Crowds at the other races have been less than spectacular. Their TV ratings, like CART's, were headed to the bottom in spite of being live on network television. Tony George has very deep pockets and apparently has no interest in getting CART and his IRL back together. The race fan has been hurt the most. Europeans are losing interest in American racing and, as the disenchantment grows, many American fans have turned to NASCAR, whose rapid growth is unprecedented and appears unstoppable. The Brickyard 400, a NASCAR race on the hallowed Indy track and an indignant slap at tradition by Tony George, threatens to outdraw the Indy 500, once the biggest sporting event in the world.

Growing more depressed as the evening dragged on, Terry and I began talking about how neither of us has much time to spend with our families. Little time exists for vacations due to the time we both devote to racing.

Terry continued to have a full operating schedule in Indianapolis and was under constant pressure from his partners to take more days of call. I continued to practice full time at the University of Miami and the University wanted me to take more call. Seeing my children and grandchildren as often as I would like was now becoming my biggest challenge. Trammell and I had immersed ourselves in racing because that's where most of our friends were and that's where we had spent most of our emotions. To say it was in our blood would have been an understatement. It was, and is, in our marrow, part of our being.

Without the occasional smell of methanol we would be certifiable. We need the diversion. Modern medicine is in a shambles. Neither of us knows many doctors happy to be practicing. The malpractice issue and governmental red tape continue to suffocate the physician, making it difficult to properly care for patients. Terry and I hope that our families understand our commitment to the sport and appreciate what we have learned from the race tracks of the world.

The future of open-wheel racing is in serious jeopardy. Not only because of the split, but because the prominence of the automobile as an icon in our society is slowly dissolving. With youth, extreme sports now rule. When we were young, a lot of us went to automobile races. They were exciting and dangerous. Today kids go to the ocean, the lake, the ski slope, the half-pipe or the motocross track. These sports offer the risks and thrills that used to be the exclusive purview of motorcycle and auto racing daredevils. I have to admit that watching a kid do a flip on a motorcycle in mid-air 40 feet above the ground is thrilling. So is snow boarding off a mountain precipice, skiing down an icy glacier and any number of other extreme and dangerous pursuits.

Most of the fans at races are now 35 and older. Sometimes I think the crowds have grown smaller only because the older fans have died off. Indy-style racing needs to attract the teens and preteens if it is to survive as a viable spectator sport. NASCAR seems the only one capable of doing that.

The cost of racing a car in a top series is too high. In 2001, to be competitive, a single-car team in CART had to have a budget of at least 11 million dollars. A two-car team almost twice as much. NASCAR was said to be higher still and Formula One has been astronomical for years. at this time Ferrari's annual budget was said to exceed 350 million dollars. We love it though, and the better part of our lives has been dedicated to saving race drivers. Open-wheel racing in America, if it is to stay alive and thrive, needs new blood and a fresh new approach. Racing still tests a man's ingenuity and his bravery. Racing drivers have evolved from the warriors of ancient Greece, the charioteers of Rome, and the fabled Knights of the Round Table.

The sport needs to recognize and market the drivers as the athletes they are. Racing needs to garner the respect shown to other, more traditional sports. Driving a racecar at speed is extremely difficult, requiring the intense concentration of a hockey goalie, the analytical thinking of a chess master, the endurance of a marathon runner, and the strength and reflexes of a boxer, not to mention the bravery of a gladiator. The drivers I know are calculated risk takers, not foolhardy thrill seekers. We have repeatedly shown that they are athletes in every sense of the word. Unlike other professional athletes, who risk little collecting millions of dollars sitting on the bench with tendonitis, a race driver risks his life every time he gets in the car. He accepts this as a fact of life. He does everything he can to protect himself, but death always lies in wait. Ernest Hemingway once remarked that there were only three adult sports, mountain climbing, bull fighting and auto racing. All the rest, he said, are just children's games.

Race drivers are driven. If they're awake and can move at all, they want to drive the racecar. We have actually had to confine them during the recovery process in order to keep them from driving some form of motorized racing machine on the sly. I have never had a driver tell me that he didn't want to drive any more after a bad crash. They only ask when they can go back.

Most spectators envy the fact that a racing driver at speed has control over his own destiny, at least for a while. If he suffers the slightest lapse in concentration, he doesn't just drop a fly ball or miss a basket, he can be savagely plastered against a concrete wall. Spectators, I think, live vicariously through the drivers they so admire. They don't want to see anyone killed or hurt. They do want to see an individual pushing the elements of risk to the maximum, cheating death in the process.

Dr. Trammell and I finally went to bed.

Chapter 36

THE GERMAN MEMORIAL CONTINUED

After Alex Zanardi's horrific crash, the race finished without further incident. I had remained by the phone since the two drivers left in their respective helicopters. I would occasionally pace anxiously about the care center, but never far from the phone. Our nurses, Liz and Sue, were still crying as they prepared to leave for England and our next race scheduled for the following weekend. The chaos around the medical center had gradually subsided and the building was largely quiet. No one had much to say. Most of the personnel remaining were absorbed in their own private thoughts. The German physicians had never seen anything quite like Alex's crash and they were awestruck. At last the phone rang!

"He's arrived alive," said the voice on the other end of the line.

The doctor in Berlin said that Alex had nearly died in the helicopter. He had needed cardiopulmonary resuscitation for a couple of minutes during the flight. My heart skipped a few beats and I broke into a cold sweat. Tears filled my eyes. Alex had made it to the hospital with no time to spare.

The doctor further explained that he had lost 75% of his blood volume by the time he arrived. From the initial impact to his arrival in the emergency room had taken 59 minutes. He was still unconscious and his blood wouldn't clot. The plasma factors needed for blood to clot had been largely depleted by the massive hemorrhage. Zanardi had been rushed to the operating room from the heliport, stopping only briefly in the Emergency Room. He was still bleeding profusely as they wheeled him into surgery. It would be a few more hours before we would know any more about his condition. He was still in grave danger, but at least he had a fighting chance. The fact that he had survived so far was a major accomplishment. Bilateral above-the-knee traumatic amputation of both legs in the field is considered a universally fatal injury.

The race finally ended. Wally Dallenbach called for a debriefing as soon as everyone was in from the track. The Safety Team gathered in a small conference room in the control tower. Faces looked worried, tired and empty. We went over the entire incident with everyone involved giving his version of what happened. In short, nothing more could have been done for Alex. The rescue was heroic. The delay at the helicopter was typical for a normal highway rescue, what the flight crew did on a daily basis. Without physicians in attendance flight medics are forced to follow a strict set of guidelines before they take off. The German medics were going by the book. Unfortunately, in this scenario time is the enemy. The definitive care Alex needed could not be given at the track. In addition to the obvious hemorrhage, he was also bleeding internally from a fractured pelvis and a liver laceration. Luckily, the helicopter crew got the message in time and he made it to the trauma center alive.

After the meeting, I went back to the medical building. It was dark, casting a further pall over the whole scene. By then almost everyone had gone. Several drivers stopped by on their way out of the race track to inquire about Zanardi. I told them he had a chance but was still in surgery and it would be several hours before we would know anything else. Jimmy Vasser, Dario Franchitti, and Max Papis were more distraught than the others. They were all close friends of his. They were angry. I gave them what little hope I could, but it didn't seem to help much.

The track graciously arranged for a fifth helicopter to fly Terry and me to Berlin. Vasser decided to go with us. He said he had to see Alex. The trip took 35 minutes. When we landed on the roof of the hospital we were greeted by Father Phil and Jon Potter. They both looked exhausted. They told us that Zanardi had just come out of the operating room. The surgeons said he was in critical, but stable, condition. I almost kneeled to kiss the floor. I hugged Father Phil and vigorously shook hands with Potter. Terry and I headed for the intensive care unit.

As we turned to go down a very large hallway, we noticed an enthusiastic young woman rushing towards us with a huge smile on her face. It was Dario's fiancée, Ashley Judd. Her personality and beauty is surpassed only by her intelligence. She grabbed me by the arm and said in a very, very professional manner:

"OK doc, he's had six and a half hours of surgery. His blood gas is good and his vitals are all normal. His electrolytes are normal and they're keeping him in a chemically induced coma for the brain swelling. He's had umpteen units of blood and blood-clotting factors and, *boy*, am I glad you're here!"

It was as good a report as I had ever received from any of my former interns or residents. Alex was going to make it!

"Thank you, my dear Ashley!"

Franchitti soon arrived, and he and Ashley, along with Jimmy Vasser, talked to Daniela Zanardi. Mrs. Zanardi had calmed down considerably by this time and was settled into problem-solving mode. She quickly made plans for the coming days. The road to recovery was destined to be a long one. Zanardi would need to stay in Germany for a few weeks, at least until he was up and around in a wheelchair.

Trammell and I had to make our own plans. We decided that Terry should fly back to Dresden to pack, pick up the wives, and if necessary bring the rental car to Berlin the next day. A lot would depend on how Zanardi did over night. I would stay in Berlin and check on him in the morning. I needed to also visit Alex Tagliani, who had been admitted for observation.

The nurses reported that Alex T had become quite despondent after being told of Zanardi's injuries. His doctors had X-rayed and scanned him from head to toe, with everything being reported as negative. His mental state was the only worry. I met with him briefly, carefully explaining that there was absolutely nothing he could have done to avoid the accident. It was amazing that he was not injured.

I then went back to the intensive care unit where I met Dr. Gerd Schroeder who would be taking care of Zanardi. Dr. Schroeder was an intensive care physician and directed a unit very similar to mine. He and I spoke the same language. He couldn't have been nicer. Together, we developed a treatment plan for Alex.

I have had previous encounters with other intensive care physicians and emergency physicians who were not only unpleasant, but downright belligerent. Confrontations with these kinds of doctors usually occurred in small-town hospitals where the local doctors felt intimidated by the CART entourage. On one such occasion in Sheboygan, Wisconsin the radiologist, the Emergency Room physician, and the hospital administrator all refused to let Terry and I into their emergency room. Rookie driver Memo Gidley had crashed big that afternoon at Road America and had been sent to the hospital for precautionary X-rays. Trammell and I were not allowed to see the films nor talk to the patient. Just the opposite, all of the doctors and staff in Berlin were secure in their expertise and extremely polite and cooperative with our foreign invasion. It was sad that in our own country so many physicians feel intimidated and are reluctant to work cooperatively with visiting colleagues.

Zanardi was in the induced coma so he had no idea who was visiting or what was happening. He was bandaged heavily, and had all of the necessary monitors in place. He appeared stable for the moment. Dr. Schroeder and I discussed his case from a critical care standpoint. We agreed on a treatment plan and timetable for the duration of the chemically-induced coma. We didn't know if he would ever wake up and if he did, we didn't know if he would be the same Alex. He had been unconscious for the duration of the extrication and the flight to the hospital. Usually this signifies a significant head injury with some residual neurological deficit if and when the patient does wake up. We agreed on 72 hours of induced coma.

During the long operation, the surgeons removed all of the dead tissue from Zanardi's two stumps and cleaned up his wounds. The monumental orthopedic question following surgery was whether or not he would ever be able to wear artificial limbs. The surgeons felt that his right leg would be suitable for a prosthetic (artificial) device but his left leg was severed just below the hip, making an artificial limb very iffy. I thanked Dr. Schroeder for his excellent care and for the tremendous cooperation. I left for the Four Seasons hotel to spend the rest of the night.

In the morning, I went straight to the hospital. Ashley was still there. She had spent the night with Daniela. Chipper as always, she gave me a full report on the patient. He had remained stable through the night with no complications. I thanked her and then went to see Tagliani.

The other Alex was still an emotional wreck. He refused to believe that Zanardi was going to survive. He was crying and very distraught. He blamed himself for the crash. I spent the next hour or so convincing him that there was no way he could have avoided it. I explained that I had watched films of the crash over and over. Zanardi had appeared from out of nowhere. There was no way to avoid hitting him. I explained how Zanardi was doing and that he was going to live. Eventually Tag began to relax and by the end of the visit he was able to smile. By a miracle, what should have been a double fatality had killed no one. Zanardi had lost his legs but not his life.

I left Berlin for England and our next race. When I arrived everyone was still quite subdued. They all wanted to go home and I was no exception. The events of 9/11 still filled the news and no one could get the images of people jumping to their deaths out of their mind. The feelings I had were the same ones I had whenever a family member or close friend had died, empty and hollow. The stress of the crash in Germany only added to our collective despair.

Leaving for America was still impossible due to the restrictions on travel, and we had another race to run. On the morning of the third day in England, Dr. Schroeder called and reported that

Alex was fully alert and neurologically completely normal. I was ecstatic! We were both surprised. Schroeder reported that shortly after the coma medicine was turned off Zanardi began to wake up. Within a few hours he was totally awake. The rapid attention he received at the scene had kept the majority of his brain cells alive. He would be limited only by the need to use artificial limbs. His brilliant and vibrant mind was remarkably intact, as was his unbridled optimism.

The outcome of the bloodiest two-car crash in CART's history was a real testament to our medical and safety program. The rapid response of the Safety Team and the quick thinking of Dr. Trammell along with a well-organized plan and state-of-the-art emergency care had saved Zanardi's life. The handling of the incident and the responses of the people involved embody all of the reasons I was still going to races after 37 years.

There is more than just the love of the sport that binds the racing community. There is also a common and intense passion shared by all of the truly dedicated. To see Ashley Judd comforting Daniela Zanardi, to see the despair on the faces of our nurses, to see and to hear the anger and concern of the other competitors, to see the utter frustration on the faces of the Safety Team when the helicopter with Zanardi finally left the track, these are the reflections of a close-knit clan.

Race teams will do whatever it takes to beat one another on the race track, but they will also do whatever it takes to help one another in a crisis. In the hours that followed Zanardi's crash, all of the good that is motor racing shone like the morning sun.

Open-wheel competition in America goes back to the turn of the century, though symbolically it probably begins with the first Indianapolis 500 in 1911. The images of Ray Harroun's toothy smile after winning that first race, or Eddie Sachs leading the Gordon Pipers' bagpipe band down the front straight on raceday mornings; the car of Duke Nalon engulfed in flames along the first turn wall, or A.J. Foyt in the pace car with Tony Hulman after winning his fourth 500; Johnny Rutherford upside down at Phoenix, Pancho Carter limping to his car in Nazareth, Pennsylvania, or Greg Moore trying to pass nearly the entire field in front of him in Portland, Oregon; Paul Tracy bullying his way through the pack on some hopelessly tight street course; or Alex Zanardi doing doughnuts for the first time after passing Bryan Herta in the dirt at the top of the Corkscrew at Laguna Seca. These are the images that define the lineage that is Indycar racing. Those of us who grew up with it, smelled it, touched it and tasted it all feel the same bond. Unfortunately, the business types who now permeate the sport don't share this same gut-centered devotion. I can only hope that the truly addicted will prevail, and that the original spirit of open-wheel competition will somehow manage to survive and prosper into the future.

Before I left Germany for England, the decision had been made that Daniela Zanardi would be the one to tell Alex about his lost legs. A few people thought that she might not be up to it. But she is made of stern stuff and insisted on it. Daniela prepared herself. She waited until Alex was fully awake and not under the influence of any medications. His response to the grim news was not one of the ones she anticipated. What Alex said, and he was smiling, was this:

"That's OK. As long as I still have you and Nicolo, everything will be just fine."

That's Alex!

Chapter 37

POST-MORTEM

C ART managed to plunge itself into bankruptcy at the end of 2003. My contract ran out at the same time. Four businessmen, calling themselves the 'Open Wheel Racing Series', bought the remains of the once mighty Championship Auto Racing Teams following the bankruptcy hearings in Indianapolis, Indiana. Many of CART's faithful employees were let go right before the Christmas Holidays. Dr. Trammell, with a year to go on his contract, and it was a well-written one, stayed on hoping for the best. The new organization did not totally live up to its promises, however, and Terry left OWRS in 2004. CART, the name, was officially changed to Champ Car and the racing continued using old equipment and the remaining teams that had not yet defected to the Indy Racing League. Their future looked "iffy" but Terry and I wished them well.

The IRL was designing a new car for its series around this same time and it was scheduled to debut in 2007. Since Terry was an expert in cockpit and seat design, he was offered a consulting agreement to work on this new project. I returned to the fulltime practice of critical care in Miami and both of us hoped we could somehow stay involved in motorsports research.

Professor Sid Watkins contacted us early in 2004 and stated that the rumored FIA Institute for Motorsports Safety was to be a reality and was touted as having a substantial budget for research projects. Terry and I, as well as Dr. Hugh Scully and Dr. John Melvin, were made Founding Fellows of the new Institute. Professor Watkins's dream of such an entity became reality and now we were all working closely with FIA engineers Andy Mellor and Hubert Gramling to produce further accomplishments in the field of motorsports safety. Professor Watkins stepped down from Formula One after the 2004 season, relinquishing that responsibility to Dr. Gary Hartstein, his longtime apprentice. Sid retained his presidency of the FIA Medical Commission and assumed the role of Chairman of the newly-formed Institute.

The Institute was not the only good news since the demise of CART. In May of 2005, I received a phone call from my old friend Emerson Fittipaldi. Emerson informed me that there was a new racing series in the works for older drivers. He explained that a man named Scott Poulter in England was putting a series together to showcase former Formula One stars over the age of 45. They wanted me to be the Chief Medical Officer. After hearing a little more of their plans, I took the customary two seconds to say yes to the idea.

Once I said yes, I began to consider what it was I was getting into. Did I really think a series like this would work? What about reflexes, vision, cardiovascular performance, stamina, heat tolerance, hearing and all the other things that tend to deteriorate with advancing age? I went to work preparing a manual and performance requirements for such a series. The first race was scheduled for South Africa in November at the old Formula One track at Kyalami, near Johannesburg.

Lynne and I left for South Africa with some real trepidation. On arrival, I had a message waiting for me from Emerson. After unpacking, I called him and he asked me to meet him in the lounge because he wanted to ask me some questions. What he really wanted was to tell me he didn't think he should race. He was visibly nervous, and the underlying anxiety was due to the tremendous amount of suffering he had undergone while recovering from his neck injury sustained in 1996. In the interim he had also survived an ultra-light plane crash with more surgery, this time on his lumbar spine.

As the conversation progressed, I sensed that Emerson was

having a mental tug of war with himself. Like the devil and angel cartoons, one part of him was still very competitive while the other part of him was reluctant to accept the associated risk. We talked for more than an hour. By the end of the conversation, the devil was winning out. That same old fire had been rekindled. I suggested to him that he should participate in the first practice session and see how he felt. I promised to help him with the HANS device and to check out his cockpit and the general safety features of the race track. Emerson accepted the plan and went off to dinner.

The next person I ran into was none other than Nigel Mansell. He and his wife Rosanne, with two of their children, were on their way to some restaurant. After saying hello to me, Nigel told Lynne that he was still suffering from a little food poisoning that he had acquired at the celebrity golf tournament the day before. He looked perfectly healthy to me. In fact, he looked to be in phenomenal shape. I'm almost certain I caught a bit of a wink. The Mansells left for dinner and Lynne and I sat down to eat as well. I picked up a newspaper on my way into the hotel restaurant and sure enough, on the front page for everyone to see, there was an article proclaiming the fact that Nigel was going to give it his all in the upcoming race, but was suffering greatly from a bout of food poisoning. Nothing, it seems, ever really changes.

The two former World Champions led the practice sessions the next day, beating the likes of Eddie Cheever, René Arnoux, Derek Warwick, Christian Danner, Andrea de Cesaris, Stefan Johansson, Alan Jones (another World Champion), Jacques Laffite, Jan Lammers, Riccardo Patrese, Hans-Joachim Stuck and Patrick Tambay. As the weekend progressed, Emerson grew more and more comfortable in the car. Driving seemed to make him shine all over. I felt reasonably secure in having convinced him to race, because he still had the skill and the desire, and he would resent it all winter were he not to compete. All of the drivers, in fact, seemed to shine. I have never, in 30 some years, seen an entire group of drivers so ecstatic. They didn't really seem to care where they qualified, they were just glad to be back in the arena. They reminded me of the kids at Christmas.

Race day dawned bright and sunny. More than 100,000 spectators showed up, 20,000 more than for the last Formula One race held there in 1993. I too was thrilled. I was back in a firesuit and all the old feelings of anticipation were there. The organizers provided me with a brand new BMW sports sedan with a trained racing driver as my chauffeur. I was blessed with two excellent paramedics to ride in the vehicle with me, and we had all the necessary state-of-the-art equipment. The medical facility was superb and the staff were friendly and competent. I truly couldn't believe it was really happening. I stopped to talk to Emerson briefly right before the start; he had that familiar look in his eyes.

The race started with all 100,000 fans on their feet. They didn't sit down for the duration of the 90 minute event. The ambient temperature was over 90 degrees and the course was full of tight twists and turns. There was little in the way of straightaways to use for a bit of a breather. Mansell started from the pole, with Emerson second. The entire field was separated by less than one mile an hour. The cars were identical and resembled the CART cars from 1999 and 2000. The engines were brand new Nicholson-McLaren Cosworths and developed over 650 horsepower. The gearshift was behind the steering wheel, the paddleshift variety. Mansell's pole speed beat the lap times of the Minardi two-seater Formula One machines being driven by former Grand Prix driver Johnny Herbert by 1.8 mph. These were real honest-to-goodness racecars.

Showing no hint of a gastro-intestinal upset, Mansell jumped into the lead at the start with Fittipaldi all over him. Patrese doggedly held on to third place, while the middle of the pack exchanged places on every lap. Johansson spun on the second lap and was narrowly missed by nearly the entire pack. Warwick was absolutely brilliant in passing more than four cars during the race. There was more passing in this race than in any Formula One race in recent memory. Toward the end, Fittipaldi tried a daring pass when Mansell made a slight mistake. Their wheels came within less than an inch of touching, with Mansell holding Fittipaldi at bay. These guys were serious!

Mansell again showed his driving prowess as he led every lap to take the first-ever Grand Prix Masters victory. Fittipaldi was second by 0.4 seconds with Patrese a distant third. The two masters had just taken over where they had left off. When the drivers got out of their cars they were all smiles, the biggest smiles on a bunch of drivers' faces that I have ever seen. After the race, Tambay vowed to get in better shape for next year. During the event, I noticed that he would do really well for a time then slow down a bit for a few laps. I asked him why, and he simply explained that he was wearing a heart monitor and when his heart rate exceeded 140 he would ease off a bit, then resume the chase when it slowed down some. Eddie Cheever, conditioned to turning only left from his recent IRL days, told me he needed to learn to turn right again. Alan Jones, not being competitive at all and withdrawing before the event, vowed to hire a trainer as soon as he got back to Australia.

The event in South Africa exceeded everyone's wildest dreams. The drivers collectively donated the prize money to Nelson Mandela's Children's Fund and all vowed to return again next year. I had been able to relax about halfway into the race. The skill of these drivers and their obvious maturity allowed me to. All the questions I had before the race had been answered. Yes, they could do it. There didn't seem to be any lack of reflexes, or vision problems, or hearing issues, or inability to stand up to the heat and duration of the event. No one collapsed at the end nor needed any assistance. These men were all seasoned veterans of the most demanding formula in motorsports. They had raced all over the world in all kinds of cars. They were the survivors.

Chapter 38

WHAT GOES AROUND COMES AROUND

S cott Poulter is a visionary. Poulter is also a doer. Poulter is
sadly too big a dreamer. Following its success in South Africa,
Grand Prix Masters held races in Qatar and in England.

The track in Qatar was a brand-new multi-million dollar facility
built primarily for the Royal family. The event was unique in that
it was an invitational. The Emir invited 2,500 of his closest friends
to attend the race. The temperature was a balmy 44 degrees C. The
race lasted 90 minutes and no one complained. Mansell won for
the second time.

The venue chosen for the race in England was the fabled track at
Silverstone. The event was the antithesis of Qatar. The day dawned
rainy and cold. The old track was treacherous, grey and damp.
Yet people came. No expense had been spared by Mr. Poulter.
Everyone with a credential received a Grand Prix Masters official
wrist watch. Hats, backpacks, and mouse pads were dispensed
as well. The hospitality facility – tent is not the correct word to
describe it – rivaled anything in Formula One. There were ice
sculptures galore, multiple open bars, and dozens of closed-circuit
television screens. A gourmet feast lay in front of the guests. After
the race, a massive concert was planned with one of England's top
entertainers. Eddie Cheever somehow won the race, his first win
against such competition. The following day the curtain dropped
on Grand Prix Masters.

Shortly after the race in England, Scott Poulter disappeared.
Rumors have him living somewhere in Canada. The organization
went into receivership. The drivers and I, among several others,

were all owed money, several thousand dollars in fact. Like so much of motorsports, what initially holds great promise soon goes up in smoke because of expectations that were too lofty, money that was spent before it became available, and management that was largely inept. Grand Prix Masters was history, a great idea gone up in smoke.

Each of the drivers went his separate way. All they took with them were their memories and their thoughts of the battles that might have been. The cars ended up in a garage outside of London, bought by two of the original organizers in the hope of a resurrection. The creditors, and there were many, were left holding the proverbial bag. Poulter was never seen again in motorsports.

My wife and I were among the most severely affected by the demise of Grand Prix Masters. Thinking an international series for the most talented drivers still fit to race could not fail, we invested in property in the state of Georgia. The lot we purchased was nestled in the foothills of the North Georgia Mountains, in a gated community, on a private lake designed specifically for tournament water skiing. Awesome, we thought. It too looked like a no-brainer. Property values were escalating almost alarmingly at the time. With what appeared to be an iron-clad contract, we decided to build a second home. The chosen builder grew up in Georgia. He looked remarkably like Kenny Rogers; a down-home, old-fashioned, country boy, the smooth-talking, innocent-appearing type who plays the good guy in western movies. He and the local bank's perky and quite attractive vice-president in charge of real estate took us for a ride. We were easy prey, living in Florida and unable to watch over the construction process. Assuring us that all was well and smiling continuously, Bo, as he was called, quickly ran up a stack of ever-mounting invoices. Once a house is started it must be finished. We were trapped. The house ended up costing more than twice what it should have. Repeated attempts to hold down costs went ignored. The bank never even inspected the property while the house was being built. Bo had been given a license to steal.

Closing on the house took place about a week before the U.S.

housing market crashed. Wall Street thieves and the major banks had allowed the development of a grossly inflated market to consume much of America. We were among the victims. It was the perfect storm. We lost the income from Grand Prix Masters, we had a second mortgage we could only marginally afford, and the value of our primary residence in Miami dropped 40%. Had things gone as expected, we would now be flying around the world with some of motor sport's most revered competitors, all expenses paid by Grand Prix Masters. We would have a second home to go to for part of the year, and, after downsizing in Miami, I would have been able to cut back at the University and enjoy part of the year in Florida and part in Georgia.

"Que' se rah se rah!"

Lynne and I were forced to regroup. Fortunately, we both had our health, our children and grandchildren were doing well, and I was still employed by the University of Miami Miller School of Medicine. The Institute in Paris was restructuring, adding a Medical Advisory Panel to oversee the development of motorsports medicine education worldwide and to better direct its research efforts. Dr. Trammell and I were actively seeking further safety innovations along with engineers Mellor and Gramling. During the period from 2003, we developed a youth helmet standard. Until its development, youth helmets were basically downsized adult versions. A three-year study produced a much more suitable helmet for children and adolescents from 6 to 17 years of age. Every major series now has professional drivers in their late teens.

Dr. Trammell worked on improving the safety of racing cars in rear impacts. I continued to champion the development of the in-ear accelerometer systems to better understand and detect concussion. And, following the near fatal crash of Felipe Massa in qualifying for the 2009 Formula One Hungarian Grand Prix, a new visor was perfected to make intrusion into the skull less likely. Professor Watkins continued to be President of the Institute, and his wife Susan wrote a play, *The Guinea Pig Club*, about the pioneering plastic surgery of New Zealand-born physician Sir

Archibald McIndoe. Professor Scully remained active as Chairman of the ICMS (International Council of Motorsport Sciences) and a prime mover in motorsports education.

While all of the above was taking place, professional open-wheel motorsports competition in the United States continued to self-destruct. Both the IRL and Champ Car continued their attempts to destroy each other. Race fans grew weary, the stands emptied, and the television audience dwindled, helped along by the worst TV sports contract ever conceived. Sponsors became disenchanted and plied their wares elsewhere. NASCAR managed to hold its own. They still used ancient technology but at least it was much safer with the addition of the HANS device and the Safer Wall not to mention a complete redesign of their cockpits by Dr. Melvin and colleagues. The concepts were developed in CART, but NASCAR claims the ideas were theirs.

Mercifully, Tony George was finally asked by his family to step down both from the IRL and the Indianapolis Motor Speedway's Board of Directors. Split into two camps for 13 years, Champ Car and the IRL in desperation embarked on an end-of-life resuscitation effort by merging. They changed the rules, agreed on the concept of a spec series, and developed into a mirror image of the original CART. Who would have thought?

Randy Barnard, the man who turned bull riding into a national phenomenon, was chosen to lead the new series. The series was finally named 'Indy Car'. In 2011 attendance at the 100th anniversary of the Indy 500 was close to the record crowd seen in 1995. TV ratings were up and sponsors were returning, if not in droves. The line on the monitor was not a flat one; there was still some activity and the rhythm seemed to be improving.

So what about me? Shortly after year's end, while working at my desk in the hospital, I received a call from a man named Chuck Aksland. Chuck, I was soon to find out, used to be Kenny Roberts' team manager. Chuck asked me if I would look at the design of a new infield care center to be built in Austin, Texas. He wanted my opinion on the layout.

"Sure," I said. "Who races in Austin?"

"Why Formula One's gonna race here," replied Chuck.

"No shit," I think I said after that.

Following a brief discussion I was invited to Austin where I was introduced to one Tavo Hellmund. Tavo, visionary, mover and shaker, as well as all-round good person, described what was in store for Austin. He also revealed that Bernie Ecclestone was a good friend of his and had actually attended his christening. He stated that the plan to develop a Formula One track in Austin, Texas began nine years earlier, conceived by he and Ecclestone when the venue in Phoenix failed. As the story goes, Bernie wanted to give Indy a try first. That attempt failed. Absent from the United States for two years, Formula One set its sights on Austin, a city for the future. Not only is it the music capital of the world, it is also home to a large number of high-tech companies, not the least of which is Dell, the computer giant. Close to Mexico and easily reached from Canada and Europe as well as South America, attendance promised to be good. In keeping with the FIA's quest for sustainability, the Circuit Of The Americas, as it was named, was intended to be the world's greenest motorsports development.

Tavo, Chuck, and I talked for more than an hour. At the end of the discussion, I was offered the job of Director of Medical Services with plans to be the Chief Medical Officer of the new United States Grand Prix. What goes around really does come back around. Shortly after accepting the job, I was asked who I would recommend to be Director of Safety. Lon Bromley accepted that assignment two weeks later. Can you guess who became Chief Orthopedic Consultant? Terry and I in fact got the band back together. It was going to be one hell-of-a ride!

Chapter 39

AS THE WHEELS TURN

Eleven years have elapsed since CART ceased operations. The first race of the newly 'merged' Indy Car series was the GAINSCO Auto Insurance Indy 300 held at the Homestead Miami Speedway on March 29, 2008. It is now May 2019. The 'hell-of-a-ride' did not go as originally anticipated.

"Where the hell are we?"

"Beats me."

Terry and I had been driving for nearly an hour and a half. We were headed to a place that was supposed to be only 45 minutes from the Pittsburgh airport. Our rental car lacked navigation, my cell phone was acting up as usual, and Terry's was packed away. He had grown tired of answering the thing. Our windshield was awash with wavelets of heavy rain. Frequent lightning made visibility scary. When accompanied by the deafening thunder, conversation was also trying. The mid-summer thunderstorm had us surrounded. Being lost was not new to us. Years before, while trying to find the race track near Dresden, Germany, we managed to drive within earshot of the Polish border. Our wives, berating us loudly from the back seat, reminded us where we stood at times like this. We were in Germany for the race where Alex Zanardi would lose both of his legs.

"These directions suck." Terry's voice was nearly drowned out by a particularly loud clap of thunder.

"We could stop and get your phone out."

"I'm not getting out in this shit!"

We inched our way onward, barely able to sustain a speed much above idle. It was now 6:00 in the evening. The plane had landed at 3:00. We were trying to find the offices of Neuro Kinetics, Inc. or NKI as it was normally known. NKI was an established business that sold vestibular testing equipment primarily to ear, nose, and throat physicians who treated vestibular dysfunction. Vestibular function is how our eyes, ears, and much of our brain determines where we are in space and time. We were going there to learn about a new device developed at NKI for the United States Navy.

This device made it relatively easy to collect the data the Navy found was important in diagnosing and following concussion. It measures ocular-vestibular reaction times, or 'OVRT' for short. Eye movements, reacting to various stimuli, are what's measured. The measurements are precise and in fractions of milliseconds. The apparatus resembles a large pair of clumsy binoculars, or goggles, held on the wearer's head by an encircling elastic strap. It's not at all comfortable, but it is capable of determining a large amount of data over a very short period of time. To test a person takes just over six minutes. Abnormal tests were found by the Navy to be linked very closely to having had a concussion, the modern scourge of sports competition that includes automobile racing. The person being examined appears to be watching a virtual reality show. Terry and I were very interested in the science as it held promise of finally having an objective way to determine when a driver had sustained a concussion and when that driver could race again.

We decided we better let someone at NKI know what had become of us. To do that required finding a workable phone. Visibility was still marginal, but we were able to make out what appeared to be a Hampton Inn adjacent to the next exit. We stopped there to make the call and get a room for the rest of the night. Howison Schroeder was the person we called. He owned NKI and had been waiting patiently for us to arrive in the lobby of his office building. We had met him during May in Indianapolis while trying out the new device doing baseline studies on the current crop of Indy Car drivers. The principal investigator of the original studies done in the Navy now worked at the University of Miami and he had convinced me that this was the way forward. His name is Michael Hoffer, a well-respected researcher in concussion and vestibular dysfunction. He arranged for us to dovetail into his study already in progress at the University. We would include the current drivers in the study. Howison wanted to meet us and was impressed that we had even heard of his product. Terry made the call.

"Hey Mr. Schroeder, you won't believe what happened to us! The flight was late, and we got lost in a severe thunderstorm trying to find your office. We've decided to stop for the night, get our phones working again, and resume the search in the morning. Hope that doesn't cause too much of a problem for you".

"No problem at all, Dr. Trammell. Get yourselves organized, call me at 7:00, and I'll guide you in. We weren't going to do anything tonight anyway except have dinner and a couple of drinks. Good night, see ya tomorrow."

"There, that's done. Let's get a room, then hit the bar next door for dinner and I could use a drink."

"Me too."

The bar doubled as a restaurant. It was moderately busy with several patrons waiting out the storm. We found a table in the corner away from most of the crowd. Every merchandising item sold by the Pittsburgh Steelers decorated the place. We settled in for much of the night. Our conversation quickly turned to a continuation of what we had been discussing for most of our flight. Unlike the old days, we now got together for only a few weekends a year to play golf. Our wives had become avid golfers and were getting rather proficient. The four of us had only been trying to play the world's most frustrating game for six years. Progress was painfully slow. We had recently played our traditional round at the 'Brickyard' the day before the 500. The Brickyard, in my opinion, is one of the finest courses in the country. Most of the holes are outside the famous oval but four of them are inside the track. It gives you a certain perspective of just how large the Speedway is. This year's race was the 100th running of the iconic event.

The crowd was memorable because it was sold out, something that had not happened since the CART years. Alexander Rossi, a phenomenal rookie, won the event.

Our conversation quickly led to a discussion of the past 10 or so years following the rapid string of changes that almost ended Indianapolis-type car racing for good. The glory years of CART were never to be again. Wally Dallenbach, perennial Chief Steward, was the main reason CART had managed to survive for 25 years. He, along with Kirk Russell, the Technical Director, held the organization together while we endured an endless string of self-serving Chairmen. International in scope, and with the best competition in motor sports at the time, CART had threatened Formula One and was light years ahead of any other series in the United States. Tragically, greed, jealousy, stupidity, envy, and incompetence arguably ended the best auto racing series the world had ever seen. CART dissolved into a quivering mass of unexciting cars, mediocre drivers, and little interest from its former fans. As fans headed for the exits, NASCAR thrived as already has been documented in previous chapters.

As previously written, Terry and I were faced with different paths to the future. I was released from the organization that replaced CART, a quickly formed group of owners who decided to take on the Indy Racing League. Terry still had a year on his contract and, as a result, became involved with CART's bankruptcy proceedings due to the fact the new organization treated his contract as an asset. As a result, it was necessary for him to retain an attorney to get free of the proceedings. He still wanted to be closely involved, however, because he was on the trail of eliminating spine injuries that were quickly becoming endemic in both Indy Cars and the Toyota Atlantic support series. Terry, always expedient, went straight to the boss. He met with Tony George, told him the issues facing the IRL, and was quickly hired as both a consultant and an on-track member of the IRL's safety team. His work with spine injuries has been virtually uninterrupted as a result. Fractures of the spine in Indy Cars have now become quite rare.

I joined the Grand Prix Masters as their Chief Medical Officer. Sadly, as described, this series lasted for only three events. Terry and I remained in close contact and I was able to join the Indy series in kind, consulting during the Indy 500. Soon, as also written previously, I became the Medical Director of the Circuit Of The Americas, or COTA. I was hired by COTA before the ground had even been broken outside of Austin. I was able to build the medical program from the bottom up. My contract was for four years, at which time I retired from that position. Dr. John Sabra, an excellent trauma surgeon in Austin, assumed the role.

After my Austin retirement, I was added to Indy Car as a consultant for severe head injury and concussion. This assignment has been terrific as it allows Terry and me to continue our research in the sport. I have also continued as a member of the FIA's Medical Commission, which meets quarterly in Paris to review and pass judgement on safety and medical issues funneled into the FIA from motorsport's entities around the world. Other members have been Professor Hugh Scully, well known cardiovascular surgeon from Canada, Dr. Paul Trafford, anesthesiologist from Scotland, and Dino Altmann, gastrointestinal surgeon from Brazil. The four of us share common opinions on much of what transpires in the world of motorsports. We remain colleagues and good friends, having been introduced to each other by the incomparable Professor of Neurosurgery, Sid Watkins.

Sid was the founder of the first traveling medical system in Europe and served as the Medical Delegate to Formula One for many years. Sid, while alive, also served as the Chairman of the Medical Commission. He sadly passed away on September 12, 2012, leaving a large void to fill in the series. The five of us always made it a point to have dinner prior to each of the Commission meetings. At dinner, we would discuss and solve many of the world's problems, not just those affecting our favorite sport. Professor Watkins customarily had the last word.

Sid wasn't the only sad passing these past several years. Big Jon Potter and Lon Bromley also died.

Jon succumbed after a long battle with heart disease. Everyone knew Jon and everyone loved Jon. He was kind hearted, a master showman, and a friend to all who wanted to be his friend. Jon was elected by the drivers long ago to be head of the Championship Drivers' Association (CDA). He retained that title until his death. He was irreplaceable as far as Terry and I were concerned due to his ability to rapidly organize everything from police escorts in foreign lands, to enabling us to gain access to medical 'off-limit areas' far and wide. Jon had many marvelous experiences while on the CART circuit but none more amazing than the time in Phoenix when he replaced the ailing songstress who was to sing the national anthem for the event. The event was being broadcast live on national television. Jon accepted the challenge and without any practice, or sheet music, he sang a beautiful rendition of our anthem, a cappella, in front of the live audience of more than 50,000 people. It was a remarkable performance.

Lon was tragically killed when a boat carrying him and Chris Pinderski, who was on vacation with his son, capsized while fly fishing on a turbulent river near Lon's home in Oregon. It was a freak accident that, in my opinion, ended the life of the best Safety Director of all time. Fortunately, Chris and his son were able to escape the treacherous waters and survive. Lon at work was always in control. Every situation we encountered, no matter how dangerous, he managed with finesse, skill, and determination. Never rattled, he was able to sort out what we were up against in a remarkably short period of time. Each of us felt secure with Lon in charge. He was the same at the track in Austin. There, he developed a crack team of medics and firemen to cover all of the motor sports events staged at COTA. He will be forever missed in the sport.

Also meeting an untimely passing was Dave Hollander, the driver of CART's 'Safety 2'. Davie was taken by cancer. A fireman by trade, his heart was forever tied to the sport of Indy car racing. He could be counted on to keep us all in good humor regardless of the circumstances. He had a great personality and did Yeoman's work tackling any job that needed doing.

Terry and I felt a great loss from the passing of all four of these talented men. We realize that we were extremely fortunate to know and to work with all of them. There remains, and always will remain, an empty place within ourselves as a result of their passing. Men like these come few and far between. Men who fit their chosen roles to a tee, not for their own benefit, but for the benefit of all who depended and relied on them to perform to the best of their ability. The rest of us were made better because of them.

As the night wore on, our mood remained dark and somber. Tragedy within the series had reared its ugly head far too often. Indy Car had become the safest it had ever been due to the combined efforts of both the researchers within the FIA and those in Indy Car, but tragedy still occurred. The FIA utilized its three research groups that had been developed by Professor Watkins to extensively study safety issues in their series, and Indy Car benefited from the combined work of Jeff Horton, Indy's Technical Director, and Terry Trammell, the Driver's Advocate, who is as much an engineer as he is a great doctor. Both men worked tirelessly to improve safety in motor sports. Many safety advancements have been made because of their combined efforts. Deaths have fortunately been much less common than in earlier decades both in Formula One and in Indy Car. Drivers can now expect to compete for several years before retiring to whatever pastime they wish to pursue.

When someone is killed, or horribly injured, it does not sit well with the drivers. They want to know why such a thing can still happen. Tony Renna, an up-and-coming young driver, was tire testing one morning at the Indianapolis Motor Speedway in 2003. He suddenly lost control coming out of turn 3, became airborne, and went directly into the grandstands at over 200 mph. He was killed instantly. Dan Wheldon, Indy 500 winner in both 2005 and 2011, died from severe head injuries he sustained at Las Vegas

Motor Speedway on October 16, 2011. He collided with another car, became airborne, and went into the debris fence where his head met a support post head on. He was also killed instantly.

Wheldon was one of the most popular drivers of the time. His death greatly affected the other drivers. They were in no mood to continue the race so it ended on that lap. They were asked to return to their cars for a possible restart, but reportedly, on the warm-up lap, some were unable to see due to their eyes being full of tears. Debris fences became a major topic of discussion and remain so to this day. No agreement on how to move forward on this matter has been reached.

Four years passed before another death shook up the Indy Car contingent. In 2015, Justin Wilson was hit in the head by a piece of debris from another car as he raced down the backstretch between Turns 2 and 3 at Pocono Raceway. At the speed he was traveling, the force was massive. He died the following day from non-survivable head injuries. A short time later, Jules Bianchi, racing Formula One in Japan, ran directly into a stationary recovery vehicle during a yellow caution period. He later died as a result.

The question of what to do about open cockpits became hotly debated. Six years earlier, Felipe Massa had been injured seriously when a spring came loose from another car running in front of him in Hungary. The spring hit the front of Massa's car then glanced toward his helmet. Massa was traveling at close to 170 mph. The spring smashed into his helmet, penetrating the visor on its left side. Massa suffered a significant brain injury, with several small skull fractures about his eye, a contusion, and a severe concussion.

Earlier that year Henry Surtees, son of the great champion, John Surtees, was hit on the head by an errant wheel from another car. Young Surtees was tragically killed as a result. After these two crashes, Formula One began to investigate in earnest a way to protect drivers better, but still retain the open-cockpit concept that defines open-wheel racing. Indy Car would start a similar quest around the same time.

The FIA's newly formed Global Institute for Motor Sport Safety, led by their chief research consultant Andy Mellor, began to develop what has evolved into the 'halo'. The halo is a very strong addition to the car. It is tubular in nature and surrounds the cockpit leading posteriorly from the head surround area. It is supported at its mid-point by a narrow post that rises from the most forward rim of the cockpit. The entire structure is elevated approximately four inches above the cockpit rim, surrounding it entirely. Not aesthetically pleasing, it does limit the ability of objects such as tires, or even an entire car that might pass overhead, from hitting the driver. The halo is built to tolerate 125Kn of force, an amount sufficient to surpass any reasonable assault on a driver who is well restrained within the cockpit. Put into use for the 2018 season, the halo likely prevented injury to a driver in two instances that first year. As a result, mandatory use of the halo was extended to all FIA categories for open-cockpit cars in 2019.

Indy Car has taken a different tack to better protect their drivers from debris or large objects intruding into the cockpit during competition. Their device is basically a shield made of a 'space age' material developed by an American company. This material is stronger than the composite material that is used in the chassis. Since it sits where a windshield might sit, it is also transparent without any distortion to the driver's vision day or night. In fact, there will likely be airplanes designed soon with parts of their fuselage made from this material, allowing a passenger to feel as if they are enjoying a magic carpet ride.

Windshields or screens aren't new to Indy Cars. They have been present off and on in various forms for many years. Bill Vukovich had a flimsy one in place when he won Indy in 1954. The 'shield' now being considered by Indy Car has been designed to deflect any approaching object such as a piece of debris, a wheel or tire, or an airborne car passing overhead. Considerable development and testing has been happening. It is anticipated that the final design will be introduced sometime during the 2019 season. Both the FIA, and the Indy Car solution, appear to be a step in the right direction to allow the drivers a much safer cockpit from which to ply their trade. No one I know who loves open-wheel racing wants the cockpits closed. To do so would destroy the look and the performance of the cars we love.

"You hungry yet?" I asked.

"Could probably eat half a cow," was the reply.

We ordered our meals and another drink. Me, a Belvedere and Terry, a Grey Goose, both on-the-rocks.

Our conversation resumed after we had consumed the reasonably good meals. Since retiring from the practice of critical care medicine in 2015 after 43 years, I have devoted much of my time and effort in understanding and treating concussion. While working in the intensive care unit at Jackson Memorial Hospital in Miami, I was mostly involved in caring for individuals who had suffered terrible brain injuries. Concussion, also referred to as a 'mild traumatic brain injury', was an injury that occurred frequently and was thought to be of little consequence less than 20 years ago. Everyone the world around used to think that a concussion was 'no big deal'. Now, of course, we know better. Too many concussions, or concussions too close together, are now known to cause serious issues later in life in some unfortunate athletes. Sadly, we too often hear about some former National Football League player who has developed a form of dementia after having played football since childhood. It has been estimated that this disease may affect 35% of American professional football players during their lifetime. Called chronic traumatic encephalopathy, this 'newer' form of dementia acts like Alzheimer's disease but is actually caused by a different protein that gets deposited into an affected person's brain. Primarily affected are the nerve tracks that transport the brain's internal messages. Terry and I have worked closely together these past few years to prevent concussion as much as possible in Indy Car. We have been quite successful. Over the past five years, Indy Car, the fastest form of closed-course racing in the world, has had only five concussions. Remarkably, no concussions have occurred over the last three years and this excellent result has occurred in spite of some very severe crashes.

The FIA has also worked to curb the incidence of concussion. Several years ago it was learned that concussions are primarily caused by the brain being put into severe, angular rotation, either by a direct blow to the head, or by the head being put into motion by other factors. The damage occurs because the brain is anchored at its base by the spinal cord but is allowed to rotate more freely as it reaches further into the skull. Simply put, if the force is large enough, the nerve tracts within the brain can be damaged by being stretched, torn, or twisted. Someone once estimated that a concussion may actually affect as much as 80% of a person's brain.

Once this mechanism of injury became apparent, the FIA worked diligently to develop a new helmet specification. Dubbed the '8860', the new helmet weighs only 2.2 pounds, considerably less than its forerunner, and that with the radio installed. For comparison, an American football helmet weighs more than twice as much. Put into motion, the old, heavier racing helmet could have a much greater effect on a driver's brain during a crash. Additionally, the '8860' was made to withstand a much greater impact. And, in order to prevent a Massa-type injury, the visor has recently been made from a material that closely resembles the windshield of a modern fighter plane, thus making penetration much less likely.

In addition to adopting the new FIA standard for their helmets, Indy Car has been gradually getting the drivers used to having their head surround fitting a bit tighter. The driver now has to actually use a little effort to push his head back into contact with the head rest. The new head surround keeps the head more in line with the long axis of the car during a violent crash. Along with the HANS device, it keeps the head from rotating as much as possible. This change has dramatically decreased the incidence of concussion. It does not, however, work to prevent concussions in every type of crash.

In 2013 Dario Franchitti had a serious crash in Houston, Texas. He lost control of the car and ran head-on into the guard rail. This impact caused his car to become airborne and to rotate violently.

In fact, it completely rotated around its vertical axis three and a half times in 1.2 seconds. Dario sustained a severe concussion as a result. Both his head and the car rotated at basically the same rate. He suffered post-concussion symptoms for over four months. Because he had sustained earlier concussions, both in racing and when a child, he elected to retire from professional motor sports. His career needed no more stunning drives. He has won Indianapolis three times, the series championship four times, and the Daytona 24 Hours, along with several other important wins during his long career. He now keeps busy with speaking engagements, television appearances, and raising a family.

The rain had finally stopped. The restaurant was less than half full. A few 'long-termers' remained at the bar. Judging by their widely spaced remarks to each other, we guessed they were most likely local truckers headquartered nearby. I swear each one had something 'Steeler' attached to him. Some wore jackets, some shirts, others caps, and who knows what they may have had on underneath. A couple of ladies, one at each end of the bar, fitted in with the rest of the appliances. Both had the vacant stare of a lost evening. Their images, reflected back from the giant mirror behind, made both of us a little sad. The bartender wore a dirty white apron with 'Steelers' embroidered on the front. I for one loved the Steelers, their big quarterback impressed the hell out of me as he defied medical science and still won ball games. It was now 11:30. We hadn't stopped talking since dessert. Morning would come too quickly.

"I sure hope we're not wasting our time on this trip."

"Me too. The Navy thinks this is the best thing so far. It's totally objective. The drivers can't game it like they've learned to do with the other tests we use. I was talking to a doctor in Miami last week who has worked with World Cup Soccer. He said they have the same issue with their players. Hoffer's sure high on this OVRT system. He was looking over some of our results and made the comment that our tracings are quite similar in a lot of respects to the ones he's seen with fighter pilots. Both the drivers and the pilots appear to have the ability to shut down much of their peripheral visual responses. A good attribute for someone traveling more than a soccer pitch a second on a narrow race track or flying at Mach 2 plus something somewhere over the world."

"That's all correct! I'm hittin' the sack, see ya in the morning."

My mind was still racing when I pulled the sheet over me. I wondered what the future held for motor sports. Some years ago I was pretty pessimistic. Electric cars were in the works, fuel was someday going to get truly scarce, kids didn't seem to give a damn about cars anymore and, when you looked at the race crowds of the world, it was difficult to find more than a few young children. In spite of my feelings back then, it seemed that racing was still holding its own.

In 2014 the FIA did indeed start an all-electric series called Formula E, with several former Formula One drivers and an occasional Indy Car driver in the field. The cars were not lightning fast, but they did put on a good show. Their biggest problem was their batteries. They could not last an entire race so the drivers had to stop and change cars approximately mid-way through the event. Crowds were good and they were adding more and more events worldwide, many in exotic places such as Paris, Rome, and Monaco.

We held a race in Miami in the first season of Formula E. It took place on the streets downtown, a similar layout to the CART race held there years earlier. I was asked to be Chief Medical Officer so it was no surprise who I chose to be the Chief Orthopedist. Terry also worked rescue on track that weekend. We learned much about electric cars. Their batteries were a bit scary as they could be a real danger if not handled properly. Difficult-to-extinguish fires and even severe explosions were possible. We learned to be very careful when handling a wrecked car. Both the driver and the rescue teams had to be cautious. Gloves had to be worn, rubber mats were used to step on, and the car had to be grounded or the battery turned off.

Fortunately, the race went without a hitch. The crowd was

excellent, and everyone seemed pumped for another race downtown the next year. However, a second race was not to be. The rumor was that the police, fire, and ambulance people wanted too much money to provide their services. Miami was so accustomed to big events that the city workers didn't really want to add any more events to their load. The series itself seems to be thriving, however, with races being held in major cities all over the world. Terry and I wish them well.

Troubling most motorsports sponsors is the fact that teenagers still don't seem to be at all enamored with the automobile and driving. I have grandchildren who didn't bother to get their licenses until they were nearly 20 years old. We have Residents at the hospital who don't drive at all. It's cheaper and less of a hassle for them to use Uber or Lift to get around town. What kids do seem enamored with is electronics. Cars have become more like rolling laptops. Rather than sports cars, as in the 50s and 60s, the favorite models now are SUVs that enable an easy escape to the outdoors.

An SUV can carry everything a young person needs to survive nowadays; backpack, food, digital movies, music, games, and the necessary gear for whatever, and much more. Extreme sports remain very popular among the younger crowd. Included are arena dirt bikes and rally cars along with extreme skiing, surfing, and backpacking. Rallycross has enjoyed great success of late especially among the under 40s.

In racing, young talented drivers, both male and female, still compete for admission to the big leagues. Drivers hoping to get into Formula One, Indy Car, and NASCAR are getting younger and younger. Recently, we convened an age-limit committee in the FIA that I served on. We suggested to the rules committee that no one under the age of 18 should compete in Formula One. At the time, there was a 16-year-old driver trying to enter. Drivers as young as 15 have competed in some NASCAR series, and I took care of a 13-year-old who had a concussion in a sprint car race in Texas. He was the only driver under 18 in the series and he was actually winning races.

I feel rather strongly that the top racing series are actually helping to inhibit their own growth. In Formula One, the car is felt by many to be 80–90% of the performance with the driver only partly affecting the outcomes. At Indianapolis, the cars went faster in the 90s than they do now. With all the safety features added in the past 10 years, plus the Safer Barrier, I would feel reasonably comfortable with the cars averaging 235 mph to perhaps greater than 240 mph on the famous oval. NASCAR, I feel, has run too slow for several years. Their most dangerous issue is 'pack racing'. The racing does appear close, but that is because the rules make it that way. Their form of racing allows the lesser drivers to keep up and mix in with the better ones. The big crashes that result are reasonably safe because they have adopted most of the safety features from the other two major series. However, unusual crashes do occur that negate some of the safety features that are normally in place. People want to see records broken, trust me. Crowds don't want to see anyone injured or killed, but they do want to see drivers challenge those risks. Risk taking gives racing drivers and other dangerous sports competitors the highest high there is, the same with engaging in any activity that invites catastrophe. Hotly contested races, driven at the maximum speeds possible, allow the rest of us to experience a tiny bit of what the drivers experience as we live vicariously through them. I am sure of that.

And lastly, tradition needs to be preserved at all costs. My family has sat in the same seats at Indy for over 40 years. We can all recite the opening ceremonies by heart. We love the noise, the smells, the anticipation, the fear that hangs over it all, and whether that weather window will smile on us again if it is needed. The Race Day diet doesn't change. It doesn't matter that carburetors are no longer used, we still need 'carb' day. Adding a big concert establishes a new tradition and that's OK. Jim Nabors is sorely missed, as is Tom Carnegie, and of course, Mr. Hulman. Their replacements carry on in fine style. The Speedway is to be commended on their success in keeping things as much the same as possible. Change is inevitable, but it can be gradual and with gentle effect on those who attend an event year after year. The traditional races like Monaco, Spa, Daytona, and Sebring seem to understand this. Newer tracks like COTA, Bahrain, and Singapore need to establish their own traditions and stick with them. Please leave Silverstone and Elkhart Lake alone!

I think motor racing will have a bright future if a few things get turned around. Records need a chance to be broken. Team performance needs to be put back into the hands of the driver. Driving race cars is an art form that dates back to the charioteers of ancient Rome. Crowds want the driver to determine the outcome, not the car. Team budgets need to be held under control. Series where only two or three teams are competitive may soon be in big trouble. That is too boring. It would also be good to see more colleges and universities with motor sports programs. Collegiate go-kart racing would be a hell of a team sport. Hybrid karts would be scientifically built, environmentally sound, and a definite challenge to young scholars. Races could be held in stadiums and practice fields on artificial surfaces. Something needs to change relatively soon as TV ratings in all series are dropping annually, crowds are generally decreasing, and press coverage has diminished. Well, I have likely gone on too long.

We met for breakfast at 5:30. It had been a short night. I asked Terry how he had slept. He said he was awake most of the night thinking about what we had discussed. His mind was always working to make new discoveries and to improve on any situation that needs to be improved. The amount of effort he has put into making racing safer for the drivers is absolutely huge. I think most of them know that, and they are very appreciative. We both consider many of the drivers genuinely good friends. We hear about what their children are up to, we attend some special family events, and we grieve during the bad times. Racing truly is a large family that transcends geography and the many different series in competition. Many times I have been approached by a driver or a crewman I don't know from a series I have never been involved with. They walk up to me, extend their hand, and tell me how much they appreciate the work I have done. It makes me feel truly gratified, happy, and rather humble to say the least. We are older now, especially me. We are still productive and continue to work to make our sport better in any way we can. Neither of us plans to stop any time soon.

Terry called Howison and was given the directions to NKI. It seemed fairly simple now that the rain had stopped and the skies had cleared. We headed north. Howison said we should be there in 25 to 30 minutes. We didn't speak much along the way as we were both deep in thought. We had discussed much the days before trying to cover more than 35 years of working so closely together. I honestly can't remember us ever having a serious argument. An occasional disagreement, yes, but it was always settled before sunset. We have experienced so much. Tragedies, triumphs, complications, special relationships, challenges that were nearly insurmountable, and a lasting and very valuable friendship.

"You know Terry. I think motor racing does have a chance to survive if the right things happen."

"I hope it does my friend. I hope it does."

AFTERWORD BY
PROFESSOR SID WATKINS

This remarkable book is a description of the struggles, dedication and vocational drive of Dr. Steve Olvey to improve medical and safety response in the sport that has fascinated him since a child.

From the early days of his apprenticeship in motor racing medicine in the '60s, the evolution and interest in developing safety features in USAC, CART, NASCAR and, latterly, IRL has been massive. The development of a core of similarly dedicated people was integral to the success of this venture in the United States. Dr. Terry Trammell, Dr. Henry Bock and their disciples joined Steve Olvey and now provide highly sophisticated response with marvellous facilities in terms of diagnostic and life-saving equipment throughout the circuits of North America.

In reaching this level of excellence, Dr. Olvey relates the difficulties of persuading circuits, promoters and finally sanctioning bodies that the development of such a system was germane to the management of many accidents and life-threatening injuries occurring in the sport.

The stamina of these pioneers to withstand the political pressures which opposed their early efforts had to be matched with great psychological fortitude to control the emotional responses in managing the many accidents and massive injuries, some of which were inevitably fatal.

In Canada, Professor Hugh Scully, Dr. Jacques Dallaire and subsequently Dr. Jacques Bouchard and Dr. Ronald Denis were facing the same difficulties. In Europe in the 60s, Jackie Stewart led the battle for safety after his experiences and his severe accident at Spa in the 1966 Belgian Grand Prix. In France, Dr. Jean-Jacques Isserman, President of the French Federation of Automobile Sport Medical Commission, was developing medical and safety protocols. In the UK, the RAC Medical Commission led by Dr. Ken Walker and subsequently Dr. David Cranston were establishing standards of excellence at British circuits. As the medical standards gradually improved focally in the 70s, in the global sense there was still a need for co-ordination on an international scale. In 1978 Bernie Ecclestone, then President of the Formula One Constructors Association (FOCA), and subsequently Jean-Marie Balestre, then President of the Fédération Internationale de l'Automobile (FIA), instigated improvements in the medical and safety response through the medium of Grand Prix Formula One Racing. The power of the Medical Commission of the FIA formed in the early 80s was fundamental in demanding sophistication in medical teams, medical centres, receiving hospitals and evacuation of the injured by a rapid response at the circuits and helicopter availability being present. As the medical sophistication spread, research into injury prevention developed and in Europe in 1994 Max Mosley, President of the FIA, formed an Expert Advisory Group initially for Formula One safety research and development. In North America, the pioneers Olvey, Trammell, Bock, Scully, Dallaire and Melvin had formed the International Council of Motorsports Sciences (ICMS) with similar goals.

In 1997 in Monaco the FIA held an International gathering of scientists, engineers, designers and doctors and it was agreed to co-ordinate the research activities worldwide. This led subsequently to the first joint meeting of the FIA and the ICMS in London in 2000 to which Steve Olvey refers in his book. Since then, in alternate years there has been a joint meeting of these organisations.

In 2003, at Max Mosley's request, the Expert Advisory Group extended its remit to include rallying and closed car racing, and in 2004 karting. At the beginning of 2004 the FIA President and the FIA Foundation decided to establish an Institute for Safety in Motor Sport and the new body was inaugurated in Paris in October 2004. The Institute is provided with a budget from the FIA Foundation and has as its core faculty the original Expert Advisory Group and in addition experts from rallying and kart racing.

The research activities of the Institute are controlled by three Commissions: Open Car, Closed Car and Karting. To this core faculty in 2005 the Institute developed and added Fellowships in recognition of the work of distinguished individuals in the world of safety and medicine. To this end, the Institute now has Dr. Olvey, Dr. Trammell, Dr. Bock, Dr. John Melvin, Professor Scully and Professor Gérard Saillant upon whose experience and expertise can now be drawn to pursue its goals.

AFTERWORD BY
DARIO FRANCHITTI

I first came to race in America in 1997. It was a bit of a baptism of fire as I crashed in my first race!

I met Steve Olvey and Terry Trammell that day. They seemed like good people but I had no idea what a major part of my life they'd share over the next 20-plus years.

During those years the safety advances have been impressive and much appreciated by the drivers, their families, teams and fans alike. The safer barrier, the HANS device, energy-absorbing seat and head surrounds, to name a few. Even the shape of the pedals and steering wheels have been changed to minimize injury. The increased understanding of head injuries has been remarkable, from diagnosis to treatment; it has moved on a great deal from 1997 (and it was really good then).

Throughout my career in America I was thankful for every one of those safety advances and I was especially thankful for Steve and Terry and their respective skills. They rebuilt me countless times. When broken bones and head injuries came, they both took care of me and got me back on track. After my last crash the team got back together one last time, unfortunately for me it was an accident too many and rather than talking about when I could get back into the car they were telling me it was over. I'm glad it was them who told me; they are my friends.

Racing is a dangerous sport and we've lost some great people along the way. This has pushed CART and Indy Car to continue to improve safety in all areas. From the safety team to the nurses and the doctors, they are a small, dedicated group and take it very personally when someone is injured or worse, so they constantly push to make things better.

INDEX

Page numbers in italics refer to photographs in the photographic plate sections

309